The hands-on guide to practical prescribing

OLIVER JONES
MA (Oxon), DM, FRCS

NANDAN GAUTAM
MA (Oxon), MRCP

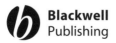
Blackwell
Publishing

© 2004 by Blackwell Publishing Ltd
Blackwell Publishing, Inc., 350 Main Street, Malden, Massachusetts 02148-5020, USA
Blackwell Publishing Ltd, 9600 Garsington Road, Oxford OX4 2DQ, UK
Blackwell Publishing Asia Pty Ltd, 550 Swanston Street, Carlton, Victoria 3053, Australia

First published 2004

Library of Congress Cataloging-in-Publication Data

Jones, Oliver (Oliver M.)
   The hands-on guide to practical prescribing / Oliver Jones, Nandan Gautam.—1st ed.
      p. ; cm.
Includes bibliographical references and index.
   ISBN 1-4051-0822-3
   1. Drugs—Prescribing—Handbooks, manuals, etc.   2. Clinical pharmacology—Handbooks, manuals, etc.
   [DNLM: 1. Pharmaceutical   Preparations—Handbooks.   2. Prescriptions, Drug—Handbooks.   QV 39 J78h 2003]   I. Gautam, Nandan.   II. Title.

   RM138.J66 2003
   615'.14—dc21   2003014051

ISBN 1-4051-0822-3

A catalogue record for this title is available from the British Library

Set in 8/9.5 Erhardt by SNP Best-set Typesetter Ltd., Hong Kong
Printed and bound in the United Kingdom by MPG Books Ltd, Bodmin, Cornwall

Commissioning Editor: Vicki Noyes
Managing Editor: Geraldine Jeffers
Editorial Assistant: Nic Ulyatt
Production Editor: Karen Moore
Production Controller: Kate Charman

For further information on Blackwell Publishing, visit our website:
http://www.blackwellpublishing.com

The hands-on guide
to practical prescribing

Contents

Abbreviations

ACE	angiotensin-converting enzyme	ECG	electrocardiography/electrocardiogram
ADR	adverse drug reaction	ENT	ear, nose and throat
AF	atrial fibrillation	ER	oestrogen receptor
AITP	acute idiopathic thrombo-cytopenic purpura	ERCP	endoscopic retrograde cholangiopancreatography
APR	abdomino-perineal excision	ET	endotracheal
		FFP	fresh frozen plasma
APTT	activated partial thrombo-plastin time	Fio_2	fraction of inspired oxygen
AV	atrioventricular	GABA	gamma-aminobutyric acid
b.d.	*bis die* (twice a day)	GFR	glomerular filtration rate
BMI	body mass index	GKI	glucose, potassium and insulin
BNF	*British National Formulary*		
BPH	benign prostatic hypertrophy	GORD	gastro-oesophageal reflux disease
BSE	bovine spongiform encephalopathy	GP	general practitioner
		GTN	glyceryl trinitrate
BTS	British Thoracic Society	HDL	high-density lipoprotein
CFC	chlorofluorocarbon	HDU	high dependency unit
CJD	Creutzfeldt–Jakob disease	HIV	human immunodeficiency virus
CNS	central nervous system		
COAD	chronic obstructive airways disease	HRT	hormone replacement therapy
COPD	chronic obstructive pulmonary disease	Ig	immunoglobulin
		IHD	ischaemic heart disease
COX	cyclo-oxygenase	i.m.	intramuscular/intramuscularly
CR	controlled release		
CSM	Committee on Safety of Medicines	INR	international normalized ratio
CT	computerized tomography	ISDN	isosorbide dinitrate
CVA	cerebrovascular accident	ISMN	isosorbide mononitrate
CVP	central venous pressure	ITU	intensive treatment unit
DKA	diabetic ketoacidosis	i.v.	intravenous/intravenously
DMARD	disease modification antirheumatic drug	IVU	intravenous urography
		LDL	low-density lipoprotein
DVT	deep vein thrombosis	LMW	low molecular weight
ECF	extracellular fluid	MAO	monoamine oxidase

MAOI	monoamine oxidase inhibitor
MDI	metered-dose inhaler
MI	myocardial infarction
MIMS	*Monthly Index of Medical Specialties*
MRSA	methicillin-resistant *Staphylococcus aureus*
NHS	National Health Service
NICE	National Institute for Clinical Excellence
NIDDM	non-insulin-dependent diabetes mellitus
NRT	nicotine replacement therapy
NSAID	non-steroidal anti-inflammatory drug
OCP	oral contraceptive pill
o.d.	*omni die* (once a day)
PAF	platelet-activating factor
Pa_{O_2}	arterial pressure of oxygen
PCA	patient controlled analgesia
PCEA	patient controlled epidural analgesia
PE	pulmonary embolism
PEFR	peak expiratory flow rate
PID	pelvic inflammatory disease
PPI	proton-pump inhibitor
p.r.n.	*pro re nata* (as required)
PST	plasma separated tube
PT	prothrombin time
PTCA	percutaneous transluminal coronary angioplasty

q.d.s.	*quater die sumendus* (four times a day)
SA	sinoatrial
s.c.	subcutaneous/ subcutaneously
SR	sustained release
SSRI	selective serotonin reuptake inhibitor
SST	serum separated tube
STEMI	ST segment elevation myocardial infarction
SVT	supraventricular tachycardia
t.d.s.	*ter die sumendus* (three times a day)
TENS	transcutaneous electrical nerve stimulation
TPN	total parenteral nutrition
TTP	thrombotic thrombocytopenic purpura
UF	unfractionated
VT	ventricular tachycardia
WHO	World Health Organization

Abbreviations used in other publications

ADR	adverse drug reactions
C/I	contra-indications
INT	drug interactions
S/P	special precautions

1: **General introduction**

What this book is about

The practical aspects of clinical pharmacology are often poorly taught. Most medical students receive a thorough grounding in the basic science of pharmacology: the classification of receptors and the mechanism of action of drugs. During clinical training, this knowledge is extended into the use of drugs as applied to disease states with more explanation of mechanism of action. In the latter part of their clinical training, medical students 'shadow' house officers and familiarize themselves with the 'hands-on' aspects of the job: clerking patients, drawing up theatre lists, taking blood samples and placing cannulae.

However, medical students are not permitted to prescribe drugs and so the practical aspects of prescribing drugs are often foreign to newly qualified doctors. Many will recall the first prescription they wrote after qualification, indeed it almost defines 'being a doctor'. For many of us, the first time we were handed a drug chart, we felt burdened with the responsibility of prescribing but ignorant of the mechanism. We knew four classes of drugs to treat hypertension but did not know which drugs (if any) a patient should take on the morning of his/her operation.

What this book is for

This book aims to address the very hands-on practical aspects of prescribing. It is not an exhaustive list of drugs, their indications, contra-indications, side-effects and dosage. Nor is it a manual of medical care. These books already exist and could not be improved by us. Indeed, this book is intended for use alongside a text such as the *BNF* or *MIMS* and not in its place. More and more hospitals are developing local protocols, hospital formularies and guidance for junior doctors. These are invaluable and should be consulted.

This book aims to give general reasonable advice on how to manage many practical aspects of prescribing. Any doubts about management should trigger consultation of texts such as the *BNF*, discussion with colleagues and pharmacists and advice from senior colleagues.

Not everything is covered and some readers may not find all their questions answered; for this we apologize. We took the problems that we had encountered, problems that our colleagues encountered and issues brought to our attention by junior members of the team and concentrated on these. There will be omissions for some readers and too much detail for others.

In general, Recommended International Non-proprietary Names (rINN) for medicinal substances are used in accordance with Directive 92/27/EEC.

2: **Practical aspects of how to prescribe**

As medical students, we are taught about drugs, how they work and when they should or could be prescribed. However, how do you actually write a prescription so that it is effective, safe and reliable? This is covered here.

In-patient prescribing

Before you start

Always check that the patient in the bed corresponds to the name on the drug chart you are holding. Always ask the patient if he/she has any drug allergies and what form the allergic reaction takes. You should not rely on the (often inaccurate) information either in the notes or written on the chart itself.

Practical prescribing

Apart from the name of the drug itself, you will have to consider the dose, the route of administration and the frequency and maximum dosage permitted. Write quantities in grams if over a gram; if less than a gram but more than a milligram, write as milligrams; if less than a milligram, write as micrograms. g and mg are acceptable abbreviations, but ug, mcg or µg are not. All may be mistaken for mg and so the full and unambiguous microgram should be used. Decimal points should generally be avoided, as they may become 'lost'. If necessary,

always precede a decimal point with a zero (i.e. 0.5 mL not .5 mL). The term units should not be abbreviated to U. However, some abbreviations are frequently and safely employed; the common ones are listed in Table 2.1.

There is a section on the front of the chart for the patient's details. Their full name, hospital number and date of birth should be written in as a minimum.

There are, broadly speaking, four ways to prescribe a drug and each has its own section on a drug chart.

1 *Single-dose drugs.* This section is usually on the front of the chart. In addition to dose and route of administration, the time and date on which the drug is to be given should be entered. An example of such prescribing would be single-dose antibiotics as prophylaxis prior to an intervention.

2 *Regular medications.* This section is used for prescribing medications that should be given on a regular basis, at the same dose and at the same time on every day. This section of the chart includes a column where the timing of doses should be stated. An example of a type of drug commonly prescribed in this manner would be an antihypertensive drug.

3 *As required medications.* The patient or the nursing staff will use their judgement on when these drugs are required. For this type of prescription, the drug dose itself and a minimum dose interval must be stated, such as 'maximum frequency every 4 hours' or 'not more than 150 mg in any 24-h period'.

Table 2.1 Common abbreviations used on drug charts. The full Latin terms are rarely used and are included only to explain how, for example, twice daily came to be abbreviated as 'b.d.'

Abbreviation	Latin term	English meaning
o.d.	*omni die*	once a day
b.d. (or b.i.d.)	*bis die*	twice a day
t.d.s. (or t.i.d.)	*ter die sumendus*	three times a day
q.d.s. (or q.i.d.)	*quater die sumendus*	four times a day
mane		in the morning
nocte		at night
p.r.n.	*pro re nata*	as required
stat.	*statim*	immediately
p.o. (or o)	*per os*	by mouth
p.r.	*per rectum*	by the anal route
p.v.	*per vaginum*	by the vaginal route
i.m.		intramuscular
i.v.		intravenous
i, ii or iii (or T, TT, TTT)		one, two or three tablets

4 *Infusions.* The quantity of drug, its reconstitution or dilution, route and rate of infusion should all be specified. Fluids may be prescribed on this section in some hospitals, although in others a separate form is used.

Routes of administration

Oral medications (given by mouth)

These are absorbed from the gastrointestinal tract and can be affected by hepatic metabolism prior to release into the systemic circulation. Some drugs may require this first pass metabolism to become active.

Some drugs need the acid environment of the stomach and will not be absorbed if there is concurrent use of antacids or acid suppressants.

Subcutaneous

This route is commonly used for vaccination. It has unpredictable absorption and is only suitable for low volumes of water-soluble agents. It has the benefit of ease of administration. Insulin is probably the most common of the regularly used subcutaneous agents.

Intramuscular

Intramuscular drugs can be rapidly absorbed. The route is useful if others are difficult. The main problems are haemodynamically compromised patients in whom peripheral muscle circulation may not be consistent. This may lead to a highly variable plasma concentration. Also, the route can be very painful and should be restricted to low volumes only. Some antibiotics can be given intramuscularly.

Per rectum

Most drugs can be formulated for rectal administration. The reason this route is not frequently used is largely social acceptance. It is invaluable in cases where oral prescriptions are not tolerated.

Buccal, transdermal

These are also viable methods. The transdermal route is useful for slow-release preparations such as glyceryl trinitrate (GTN) or hormone replacement therapy (HRT). The buccal route is for rapid absorption and fast-acting effects. Both routes avoid first pass metabolism.

Inhalation

This route is largely limited to the treatment of airways diseases including infections. In resuscitation situations, adrenaline (epinephrine) can be given via endotracheal (ET) tubes into the lungs.

Topical

Used where high local concentrations of drug are needed with few systemic side-effects.

Drug preparations

Some drugs are formulated to be slow release and the mechanisms for this vary. Some are coated to be slowly broken down, others have a more complicated system. The 'enteric coating' of drugs that might otherwise be directly irritating to the gastric mucosa is rarely useful. If any slow-release drug is chewed or crushed, the slow-release function may be destroyed and this is very important if using a nasogastric tube.

The new patient

Routine admissions

For many junior doctors, clerking of routine or emergency admissions to hospital forms a large part of their daily workload. Patients who are routine admissions to hospital should generally continue their drugs, which should be written onto their drug charts, unless these are likely to interfere with their reason for admission (beware particularly anticoagulants and interventional procedures or surgery).

It is important to ask every patient which medications he/she is taking, their doses, frequencies and routes. If the patient has brought the medications themselves, it is often useful to confirm with the patient which medications are being taken. It is worth remembering that, although a medication may be prescribed, this does not mean that it is taken by the patient. Furthermore, what is written on the box of tablets may not correspond to how the patient actually takes the drug. Other sources of information include computer printouts and handwritten lists. Relatives (especially carers) may also be reliable sources of information. A telephone call to a patient's general practitioner

(GP) usually resolves any residual uncertainties.

Emergency admissions

In general, patients admitted as an emergency should also take their regular medications as described above. However, the following additional issues should be considered.

1 Their emergency admission may have been contributed to by some aspect of their drug regimen, e.g. digoxin toxicity.

2 Symptoms such as vomiting may mean some oral medications are not appropriate.

3 The institution of an acute or new therapeutic regimen, such as nebulized bronchodilators, might render aspects of their usual drug regimen temporarily or permanently redundant; e.g. b.d. salmeterol with 4-hourly salbutamol.

4 The likely outcome of their admission may modify their drug regimen. For example, patients likely to undergo surgery may be kept 'nil by mouth'. Drugs could be given via another route, such as intravenously but, in practice, anaesthetists will often be keen that important drugs, such as antihypertensives, are still given with a sip of water.

Out-patient prescribing

When writing a prescription for medications for the patient to take away from the hospital, the general principles for in-patient prescribing apply. In many hospitals, different out-patient prescription scripts are used, depending on whether the medications are to be collected from the hospital or practice pharmacy, or whether the prescription is to be collected from an 'outside' pharmacy. Your pharmacist and/or colleagues should be able to tell you the local policy. There are additional considerations, which centre on the issue of length of treatment course. Choices include:

1 A single course of treatment only. The out-patient script should state this clearly, e.g. with the words '1 week only, then stop'.

2 A medication that should be taken continually, such that when the course as dispensed by the prescription is finished, the patient continues the drug treatment through obtaining a further 'repeat' prescription. In such cases, it is important that the GP (via discharge summary or clinic letter) and the patient (by verbal advice or copy of the correspondence to the GP) are aware that the treatment must be continued. It is poor practice for 'repeat' prescriptions to be endlessly given without review.

3 Occasionally, external prescription sheets will be needed but these should be written containing the same detail. The senior nurse will be able to locate these for you.

Controlled drugs

Out-patient prescriptions for controlled drugs have special requirements. The following are legal requirements that must be included on the prescription:

1 The prescriber must sign and date the prescription in his/her handwriting.

2 The address (hospital or practice) of the prescriber.

3 The handwritten name and address of the patient in indelible ink.

4 The form and strength (as appropriate) of the preparation.

5 The total quantity of the preparation in both words and figures, e.g. 'Total amount of morphine: 420 g (four hundred and twenty grams)'.

Brand name or generic name?

It is generally better practice to use the generic (non-proprietary) name of a drug. The pharmacist may choose to dispense whatever is available in the pharmacy, saving himself/herself and the patient time. It is also common practice for cheaper formulations to be substituted, when available. Some drug formulations affect the bioavailability of active agent and in such cases prescribing by brand is acceptable, e.g. lithium.

Further considerations

If in doubt, ask your colleagues or the hospital pharmacist. Accurate prescribing and neat handwriting minimize any confusion. They also reduce the frequency of bleeps to you from pharmacists and nursing staff. You might also consider, in all your patients, prescribing a number of additional drugs on an 'as required' basis. These additional drugs might include analgesics, night sedation, antiemetics and nebulizers. This may prevent a phone call from a nurse able to manage a patient but powerless to give them the drug they require. However, the indiscriminate and careless prescribing of these drugs should be discouraged.

3: How to use the British National Formulary (BNF) and Monthly Index of Medical Specialties (MIMS)

British National Formulary

The *British National Formulary* (*BNF*) is jointly published by the British Medical Association and the Royal Pharmaceutical Association under the authority of the Joint Formulary Committee, which in turn seeks advice from a panel of experts. It may be found on the web at http://BNF.org. It is published twice a year.

Using the *BNF*

Information about a specific drug

The *BNF* has a comprehensive index that provides the quickest route to locating a drug. Both brand names and generic names are listed. While the *BNF* is comprehensive, inclusion of a drug does not imply that the organizations and committees behind the book endorse the drug. Indeed, drugs considered less suitable are marked with a symbol ◢. However, the BNF may not list those medicines promoted for purchase by the public.

All drugs are listed in identical fashion as shown in the box on p. 8. Unlicensed indications are included for some drugs (e.g. GTN ointment for anal fissure), but where this occurs, it is clearly stated.

Cautions and contra-indications for each drug may be found in the Appendixes at the end of the *BNF*. Appendix 1 is an alphabetical list of drug interactions, where the symbol ● denotes a potentially serious interaction. Reference is also frequently made to Appendixes 2 and 3, which give further information on prescribing for patients with hepatic and renal impairment, respectively, while Appendixes 4 and 5 advise on drug prescribing in pregnancy and to patients who are breast-feeding.

Background to a clinical condition and therapeutic options

The heart of the *BNF* comprises 15 chapters, listed on the contents page, of conditions, drugs and preparations divided by organ (e.g. cardiovascular system) or medical condition (e.g. infections). At the beginning of each section, there is usually a concise summary of the clinical condition, the pharmacological options and the weight of evidence for relative drug efficacy. Individual drugs are listed in sections, with others similar either in chemical structure or clinical indication. This information can be useful in confirming the suitability of the drug that has been chosen, but also on occasion redirects the prescriber to a related alternative better for the specific indication in question.

Standard format for listing drugs in the *BNF*

[PoM] refers to prescription only medicines for drugs only available on medical or dental prescription, while [CD] denotes a controlled drug subject to restrictions in manner of prescribing and dispensing. [NHS] means that the drug cannot be prescribed under the NHS.

DRUG NAME ◢

Indications: details of use and indications
Cautions: details of precautions required (with cross-references to appropriate Appendixes) and also any monitoring required
Counselling: verbal explanation to the patient of specific details of the drug treatment
Contra-indications: details of any contra-indications to use of the drug
Side-effects: details of common and more serious side-effects
Dose: dose and frequency of administration (max dose); CHILD and ELDERLY details of dose for specific age group
By alternative route, dose and frequency

Approved name (Non-proprietary)
[PoM]
Pharmaceutical form, colour, coating, active ingredient and amount in dosage, form, net price, pack size = basic NHS price. Label: (as in Appendix 9)

Proprietary name (Manufacturer)
[PoM] [NHS]
Pharmaceutical form, sugar free, active ingredient mg/mL, net price, pack size = basic NHS price. Label: (as in Appendix 9)

Excipients: includes clinically important excipients or electrolytes
Note: Specific notes about the product, e.g. handling

Generic vs. brand name prescribing

Prescribing generically allows the pharmacist to dispense what is available in the pharmacy, increasing the likelihood of the patient being able to start treatment immediately. The pharmacist may substitute cheaper formulations if appropriate. It is worth noting that the prices listed in the *BNF* do not correspond precisely to the cost to the National Health Service (NHS), nor do they represent the cost of private prescriptions or of purchasing the drugs over the counter.

Additional information in the *BNF*

There are a number of other pieces of information in the *BNF*. These include:
1 notes for prescribing in children and the elderly;
2 permitted and prohibited substances in sport;
3 prescribing in palliative care;
4 treatment of overdose;
5 immunization and antimalarial advice for travellers, with useful contact numbers; and
6 protocols including algorithms for the

treatment of acute and chronic asthma as published by the British Thoracic Society, summary of fitness to drive guidelines for epileptics and information on prophylaxis for patients at risk of endocarditis undergoing interventional procedures.

Monthly Index of Medical Specialties

The *Monthly Index of Medical Specialties* (*MIMS*) is independently written and describes itself as a guide for GPs.

Using *MIMS*

Information about drugs and clinical conditions

In a similar fashion to the *BNF*, *MIMS* can be used either to seek information on specific drugs (by generic or brand name) or on clinical conditions. Again, it is possible to look at specific clinical conditions and examine a listing of appropriate drugs.

The general layout for drugs listed in *MIMS* is as shown in the box below.

Standard format for listing drugs in *MIMS*

DRUG NAME Company name

Type of drug. Constituents of drugs, price

INDICATIONS: Details of use and indications

ADULTS: Dose for adults

CHILDREN: Dose for children

C/I: Details of contra-indications

S/P: Special precautions/conditions where special attention is required

INT: Drugs which may be affected by or affect other drugs

ADR: Most frequently seen adverse effects or most serious rarely seen adverse effects

4: Drug interactions

Drug interactions are both common and probably under-recognized. They are listed in Appendix 1 of the *BNF*. Ward pharmacists will guide you through the important interactions and will, it is hoped, pick up any patients' drug interactions that you have missed, but it is prudent to look in the *BNF*, especially if prescribing a drug for the first time.

Knowledge of a drug interaction should not necessarily deter you from prescribing two drugs together. Often, all that is needed in such circumstances is closer clinical management or adjustment of dosage. Furthermore, drug interactions may even be used therapeutically, as in the treatment of poisoning. This chapter cannot be comprehensive in its tackling of such a large subject, but some of the principles are discussed.

Types of drug interactions

In general terms, there are two types of drug interactions: 'antagonism' is when the action of one drug opposes that of another and 'synergism' is when the effect of the co-administration of drugs is additive. The combination of two drugs may be more than simply additive and when this occurs it is known as 'potentiation'.

Drug interactions may be divided into three main types: pharmaceutical, pharmacodynamic and pharmacokinetic.

Pharmaceutical interaction

This is the interaction of drugs on a chemical non-pharmacological level. One such example is the formation of a complex between thiopental (thiopentone) and suxamethonium, which cannot therefore be mixed in the same syringe. Simple strategies should reduce the risk of this type of interaction, and include giving drugs as bolus injections where possible, avoiding the mixing of drugs prior to administration except when this is known to be safe (inevitably, many drugs have to be reconstituted in dextrose or saline) and making up infusions immediately prior to use. Lines should be flushed after each use.

Pharmacodynamic interaction

This is the increase or decrease in the effect of one drug without an effect on the drug concentration at its site of action. This is often predictable from a knowledge of the pharmacological mechanism of action of a drug and often occurs through competition at either receptor site or by an action on similar physiological systems. An example of this type of interaction is that between loop diuretics and digoxin. Loop diuretics lower plasma potassium and this reduces competition between the glycoside and potassium for the sodium–potassium pump in the heart muscle. The consequent increased glycoside binding enhances the risk of arrhythmias.

Pharmacokinetic interaction

This is the increase or decrease in effect of one drug through alteration of the drug concentration reaching its site of action by a second drug. There are four aspects of drug pharmacokinetics that may be affected: absorption, distribution, metabolism and excretion. This type of interaction may be difficult to predict and the severity of interaction (in contrast to pharmacodynamic interactions) often differs markedly between patients.

Absorption

This occurs when two drugs form an insoluble complex (seen sometimes with antacids and prednisolone) or because one drug alters gut motility, as seen with drugs such as loperamide or metoclopramide, and affects the time available for drug absorption to occur. This interaction is sometimes exploited usefully as when lidocaine (lignocaine) is combined with adrenaline for subcutaneous local anaesthesia. The vasoconstrictor effect of adrenaline reduces absorption (and hence indirectly redistribution and metabolism) of lidocaine, prolonging the anaesthetic effect of the latter drug.

Distribution

This type of interaction frequently occurs between two drugs that are extensively protein bound in the plasma. One drug may be displaced from its protein-binding site by a second. This type of interaction is often less important than might at first be considered because just as it is the free drug that accounts for the pharmacological action, it is this same fraction that is available for redistribution and metabolism, which usually restores free levels. Thus, most serious interactions are seen when displacement from plasma proteins occurs in addition to other effects such as inhibition of drug metabolism. An example of this is sodium valproate, which not only displaces phenytoin from plasma proteins but also reduces the rate at which it is metabolized.

Metabolism

This most frequently occurs when one drug affects liver enzymes such that the metabolism of a second is changed; e.g. phenytoin is an enzyme-inducing drug and may increase metabolism of the oral contraceptive pill (OCP). The resultant reduced plasma levels may result in pregnancy. Enzyme inhibitors also exist. The most common drugs in this category are those with an action that includes inhibition of isoenzymes of cytochrome p450, e.g. cimetidine and erythromycin.

Excretion

This is most commonly seen in those drugs sharing a common transporter mechanism in the kidney. An example of this is the lithium accumulation seen in patients treated with concomitant diuretics.

Table 4.1 Some commonly occurring drug interactions amongst drugs prescribed for similar clinical or physiological indications.

Drugs	Clinical effect of interaction
Digoxin and loop/thiazide diuretics	Digoxin toxicity, cardiac arrhythmia
Theophylline and beta-adrenoceptor agonists	Cardiac arrhythmia
ACE inhibitors and potassium-sparing diuretics	Hyperkalaemia
Phenytoin and sodium valproate	Phenytoin toxicity
Verapamil and beta-adrenoceptor antagonists	Bradycardia, asystole, heart failure
Lithium/MAO inhibitors and SSRIs	Serotonin syndrome

ACE, angiotensin-converting enzyme; MAO, monoamine oxidase; SSRI, selective serotonin reuptake inhibitor.

Identifying possible drug interactions

Drug interactions may manifest in a number of different ways, including lack of effect of a newly introduced drug or clinical deterioration in the patient. They are more likely in those patients taking many drugs simultaneously (especially, therefore, the elderly and seriously ill). Patients with hepatic or renal impairment are also at increased risk as metabolism and excretion are likely to be compromised.

Certain types of drugs are more likely to trigger clinically important interactions, particularly those drugs with a narrow therapeutic index (a small change in drug concentration resulting in a substantial change in clinical effect). There are three types of drugs that should alert you to the possibility of drug interactions:

1 Drugs that are bound to plasma proteins. Addition of a second drug that is also protein bound may displace the first drug from these protein-binding sites and increase free plasma concentrations.
2 Drugs that affect the metabolism of other drugs. This may occur through a number of different mechanisms but commonly involves a drug increasing or decreasing enzyme activity with resultant effects on the plasma levels of a second drug.
3 Drugs that affect renal function and alter the renal excretion of other drugs.

Important potential drug interactions

There are a number of drugs that are used for treating the same disease or condition which interact. Some of these are listed in Table 4.1.

5: **Monitoring of drugs, overdose and toxicity**

What is therapeutic drug monitoring?

Therapeutic drug monitoring is a process by which the blood concentration of a drug is maintained at a therapeutic level. It involves assaying for the drug or its metabolites at various points on the dosing schedule. Certain drugs (or their clinical effect) require close monitoring. If the clinical effect can be readily measured (e.g. heart rate, blood pressure), the dose of drug can be adjusted to response. This is not the case for drugs that are used to suppress overt symptoms such as seizures, depression and transplant rejection.

Measurement of the concentration may be needed for any drug that has:
1 a direct relationship between its concentration and the therapeutic and adverse effects;
2 a narrow therapeutic window; or
3 a therapeutic effect that is difficult to interpret and must be extrapolated from the concentration.

When to carry out drug monitoring

Therapeutic levels are based on the steady state concentration and, in most cases, this will be obtained after five half-lives of the oral dose. If loading doses have been given, steady state will be achieved faster.

Sampling at one point (the same every time) in the dosing schedule is usually enough; the time at which there is least variability is the pre-dose or trough concentration. For drugs with short half-lives in relation to the dosing interval, samples should be collected pre-dose. For drugs with long half-lives (e.g. phenytoin), samples collected at any point will be adequate. Certain drugs (e.g. digoxin) have a distribution phase and sampling should be after this (6 h later). For some drugs, both peak and trough levels are useful (e.g. vancomycin).

Values obtained can only be interpreted in the context of the individual situation. The laboratory will help to establish or revise the dosing schedule with these in mind.

1 Time of sample in relation to last dose or next dose and dosing schedule: peak or trough?
2 Duration of treatment with the current dosage. Has steady state been achieved?
3 Age, gender and weight affect volumes of distribution and other aspects of pharmacokinetics.
4 Other drug therapy. Pharmacodynamics will be affected and interactions accounted for, such as protein binding, metabolism and clearance.
5 Relevant disease states. Renal or liver dysfunction will affect dosage.

Dose forecasting is a system by which future plasma concentrations can be extrapolated from current values. It is based

Table 5.1 Therapeutic levels for some commonly used drugs.

Drug	Therapeutic level (adults)	Sample carrier	Sample time
Digoxin	1–2 nanomol/L (0.5–2 mg/L)	SST/PST heparin	6–8 h post-dose
Phenytoin	40–80 mmol/L (10–20 mg/L)	SST/PST heparin	At any point
Theophylline	55–110 mmol/L (10–20 mg/L)	PST heparin	Pre-dose
Carbamazepine	35–50 mmol/L (5.0–12 mg/L)	SST/PST heparin	Pre-dose
Gentamicin	Trough < 2; peak > 5 (t.d.s. dosing)	SST/PST heparin	Pre-dose or 2 h post-dose
Vancomycin	Trough 5–10 mg/L	SST/PST heparin	Pre-dose
Lithium*	0.5–1.0 mmol/L	SST	12 h post-dose

PST, plasma separated tube; SST, serum separated tube.
* Do not use a lithium heparin tube for lithium assays.

on average populations who are otherwise physiologically stable. This method is inexact but does have the benefit of infrequent sampling (Table 5.1).

For gentamicin, it has become increasingly common to have a once daily regimen followed by daily checks of plasma levels before further doses are given. Local policy regarding antimicrobial protocols should be sought.

Management of drug overdose and toxicity

The treatment of drug overdose and attempts at deliberate self-harm forms an important part of emergency medical therapy. There are a number of principles of treatment common to any episode of drug toxicity or overdose.
1 Stop the drug.
2 Stop further absorption. Consider activated charcoal.
3 Aid elimination of the drug. Consider charcoal, fluids and diuresis.
4 Resuscitate and correct immediate problems. Consider reversals, fluids and supportive measures.

5 Prevent progression. Antidotes, where available, may be used.
6 Surveillance for delayed effects with monitoring in hospital.

The emergency treatment of poisoning in the *BNF* gives treatment algorithms for common toxins. The National Poisons Information Service gives up-to-date advice on any toxicology-related subject. It is good practice to consult with this service in all but the most common cases (Table 5.2). You will be expected to provide your details and those of your institution, the patient's details and which agents he/she is believed to have taken. They will provide verbal (or faxed, if requested) advice from their database regarding therapy. This service is linked to drug surveillance systems (see Chapter 6).

The telephone number for the National Poisons Information Service is 0870 600 6266. TOXBASE is an online version which gives general information and is accessed via www.spib.axl.co.uk

Table 5.2 Management for commonly taken drugs.

Minimum toxic dose	Special considerations	Antidote therapy
Paracetamol*		
10 g ingested (150 mg/kg), whichever is the smaller	Lower toxic dose in liver damage or high alcohol intake or recent previous overdoses. Watch INR for at least 3 days after overdose and continue therapy until consistently below 1.3	*N*-Acetylcystine (i.v. in 5% dextrose) is effective up to and possibly beyond 24 h. 150 mg/kg in 200 mL over 15 min, then 50 mg/kg in 500 mL over 4 h, then 100 mg/kg in 1000 mL over 16 h, followed by 100 mg/kg in 1000 mL over 24 h until therapy ceases
Aspirin		
Plasma level 3.6 mmol/L in adults or 2.5 mmol/L in children	Renal function, salicylate and pH monitoring essential. Beware of hypoglycaemia	Activated charcoal is useful but patient will be nauseated. Fluids, correction of acid–base disturbances and haemodialysis are mainstay. Alkaline diuresis is no longer advised but may be needed if facilities for dialysis not available
Beta-blockers		
	Cardiogenic shock probable so HDU-type environment needed	3 mg atropine i.v. to treat bradycardia if symptomatic. Glucagon 100 micrograms/kg i.v. and inotropic support, as required
Amphetamines		
Any	Psychiatric disturbances, autonomic instability especially temperature, cardiovascular compromise all seen. May mask true cerebral irritation or evidence of encephalitis	Full supportive therapy needed. Benzodiazepines can help in early stages. Activated charcoal can be used acutely. Dantrolene (1 mg/kg) if hyperpyrexial
Opiates		
	May have effects that continue to manifest late	Naloxone, initially 400 micrograms and up to 2 mg, as repeated i.v. bolus or as continuous infusions (2 mg in 500 mL of dextrose starting at 50 mL/h and titrated to response)
		Can be given as deep i.m. injection

continued on p. 16

Table 5.2 (*continued*)

Minimum toxic dose	Special considerations	Antidote therapy
Benzodiazepines		
	Can precipitate convulsions if overdose followed therapy for seizures	Flumazenil 200–500 micrograms as initial bolus followed by i.v. infusion of 100–400 micrograms/h
Tricyclic antidepressants		
	Variable cardiovascular and neuropsychiatric symptoms. Arrhythmias can be fatal	Activated charcoal is useful. No antidote but very close monitoring and supportive therapy. Airway may become compromised with a high risk of aspiration

HDU, high dependency unit; i.m., intramuscular; INR, international normalized ratio; i.v., intravenous.
* A normogram of plasma decay is available in the *BNF*. Treat high-risk patients immediately. Do not wait for levels.

Activated charcoal is only really useful if taken within 1 h for most drugs. It is also used in cases of active elimination such as carbamazepine, theophylline and quinine. Gastric lavage is no longer recommended in most cases but, if used, the airway should be formally secured or the patient fully alert.

6: Adverse drug reactions and allergies

An adverse drug reaction (ADR) can be defined as an unintended unfavourable reaction to a drug given in an appropriate dosage and route for a correct indication. ADRs may be divided into a number of different categories, listed in Table 6.1 [1].

Types A and B are the most common ADRs. Type A reflects the interaction between the patient and the drug and is dose-related. These effects occur in many patients and are a manifestation of the mechanism of action of the drug. By contrast, type B reactions occur only in susceptible individuals and are not dose-related.

Frequency of drug reaction

ADRs are common. In a recent single practice study, GPs estimated that the presenting symptom of 1.7% of their consultations over a 6-month period was a manifestation of an ADR [2]. Furthermore, it is likely that 2–6% of hospital admissions are for ADRs [3]. Both these figures may even underestimate the true incidence.

Assessing likelihood that an adverse drug reaction has occurred

An ADR should be considered in any patient taking prescribed or over-the-counter medications; however, they are more common in young and middle-aged women. Assessing the likelihood of an ADR involves taking a careful and detailed history about clinical symptoms and their timing in relation to drug exposure. ADRs may occur immediately, and typically these types of reactions are anaphylaxis, bronchospasm and angio-oedema. Later reactions are also seen, although these are more commonly rashes and haematological changes (e.g. neutropenia or thrombocytopenia). Further clues about the relation of an adverse event to a particular drug may be obtained when the timing of peak plasma drug concentration is considered. There may be a history of previous exposure to the drug. Finally, there is also the option of the reintroduction of the suspected drug. This may be of long-term benefit to the individual, especially for those in whom alternative pharmacological options are limited, but should be done with great care.

Management of a suspected adverse drug reaction

For type A reactions, the management is simply reduction in dosage or withdrawal of the medication altogether. By contrast, type E reactions require reintroduction of the drug and more gradual withdrawal. By the time a type C or D reaction occurs, it may be

Table 6.1 Classification of adverse drug reactions.

Type of reaction	Mnemonic	Features
A: dose-related	Augmented	Related to pharmacology (toxic effect or side-effect, e.g. digoxin toxicity)
B: non-dose-related	Bizarre	Unrelated to pharmacology: idiosyncratic (e.g. malignant hyperthermia) or immunological (e.g. penicillin rash)
C: dose- and time-related	Continuous or chronic	Related to cumulative drug use (e.g. NSAID-induced renal failure)
D: delayed effect	Delayed	Apparent only some time after use of drug (e.g. thalidomide in first trimester and phocomelia limb defects)
E: withdrawal	End of use	Related to discontinuation that is too abrupt (e.g. Addisonian crisis after steroid withdrawal)

irreversible or at best only partially reversible on drug withdrawal.

Type B reactions are uncommon, unpredictable and show high morbidity and mortality. The first step is always the immediate withdrawal of the drug. If the reaction is mild, no further intervention may be necessary. Urticarial rashes and, to a lesser extent, non-urticarial rashes may be treated with antihistamines, such as chlorphenamine (chlorpheniramine), and an adrenocortical steroid. In more severe cases, these drugs may be given intravenously or intramuscularly. If angio-oedema develops with threatened laryngeal oedema, adrenaline should be considered (see below).

Anaphylaxis

Anaphylaxis is a medical emergency. Senior help should be summoned, including an anaesthetist.

1 The patient should be positioned flat, with feet raised and airway secured. Oxygen should be administered via a face mask.

2 0.5–1.0 mg adrenaline should be given as first-line therapy, by the intramuscular route (equivalent to 0.5–1.0 mL of 1 : 1000 adrenaline).

3 Repeated adrenaline administration can be performed every 10 min according to cardiovascular parameters and clinical improvement. Chlorphenamine (10–20 mg) should also be administered by slow intravenous injection, and hydrocortisone (100–300 mg), although the onset of action of the latter may not occur for several hours.

4 Further deterioration may necessitate intravenous fluids, nebulized beta$_2$ agonists and intubation or tracheostomy.

Subsequent management

Avoidance of subsequent exposure to the drug is clearly important and patient education is very important in this regard. It is worth considering that the second exposure to the drug (especially for type B reactions) may be more severe than the first.

In rare cases, desensitization should be considered. This is particularly appropriate for patients who have had immunoglobulin E (IgE)-mediated reactions to penicillin and require the drug for treatment of serious infections such as meningitis or endocarditis. This may, in theory, be carried out orally or intravenously, although the former is probably preferred as it less commonly results in serious life-threatening reactions. This is a specialist field and desensitization should only be undertaken in specialist centres.

Reporting of an adverse drug reaction

Although all drugs are evaluated prior to marketing (Phase I–III trials), ADRs either of low frequency or found only in subgroups of patients may not be detected until post-marketing surveillance (Phase IV). Part of that surveillance system in the UK requires doctors to report any suspected adverse effects to the Medicines Control Agency by using the yellow cards at the back of the *BNF*. An isolated minor adverse reaction will only become significant if many similar reports are made, but a possible major or fatal event will trigger an investigation at the first report. It is important therefore that all doctors take an active role in submitting such data.

Recently marketed drugs, identified in the *BNF* by an inverted black triangle, should have all suspected minor or major ADRs reported.

Further post-marketing surveillance is carried out by various agencies who contact doctors directly for information.

> Every unexpected adverse reaction should be investigated and usually reported by the yellow card system.

References

1 Edwards IR, Aronson JK. Adverse drug reactions: definitions, diagnosis and management. *Lancet* 2000; **356**: 1255–9.

2 Millar JS. Consultations owing to adverse drug reactions in a single practice. *Br J Gen Pract* 2001; **51**: 130–1.

3 Pirmohamed M, Breckenridge AM, Kitteringham NR, Park BK. Adverse drug reactions. *Br Med J* 1998; **316**: 1295–8.

7: **Prescribing in children**

General issues

Using the well-worn phrase, children are not just 'little adults'. The differences are both in the function of their body systems and their constituents.

Dosage

The *BNF* or a specialized paediatric formulary will confirm that the drug you are prescribing is licensed for children and will give suggestions on dosage and route of administration. If in doubt, it is reasonable to check with your ward pharmacist, but for more specialist prescribing close liaison with a paediatrician may be necessary. Many drugs used in children, however, are not licensed for paediatric usage. Scaling down of the dosage to paediatric levels tends to be based on body surface area rather than body weight.

Routes of administration

Whenever possible, medications should be given orally, either in liquid or soluble form, and many older children are capable of taking tablets. In surgical patients, who are nominally nil by mouth, it is almost always acceptable for them to take oral medications with just a sip of liquid. If a child is prescribed a liquid medication, it is important always to state the strength of solution and the amount to be taken. Many of these liquid preparations contain large amounts of sugar, which may be an issue in diabetics and may promote dental decay in patients on long-term treatment.

Neonates and infants have relatively little skeletal muscle and fat and therefore intramuscular and subcutaneous administration tends to result in unpredictable plasma drug levels. These routes are therefore generally avoided, with intravenous or rectal administration being preferred when the child is unable (or unwilling) to take oral medications.

Pharmacokinetics

Absorption

Oral absorption in children is broadly similar to that seen in adults. Transdermal absorption is often very efficient, as babies and children have well-hydrated skin. Transdermal absorption may be further increased in children with excoriated or burnt skin, but with occasional reports of toxicity.

Distribution

Young children, infants and neonates have a higher percentage of total body water, although in reality this has little overall effect on drug levels as it is cancelled out by other differences such as rate of elimination. Of greater significance is the lower plasma albumin concentration and decreased albumin-binding capacity of drugs. In neonates, the blood–brain barrier is more permeable to drugs than in adults, which explains why children are more susceptible to many centrally acting drugs.

Metabolism and excretion

The enzyme systems in the liver responsible for drug inactivation are present in the neonatal liver but are less effective. This is particularly true of the oxidative and conjugative systems.

Renal tubular function and the glomerular filtration rate are both decreased in neonates, taking approximately 6 months to attain adult values (relative to body surface area). Therefore, drugs and their metabolites eliminated by renal excretion tend to accumulate in this group. Aminoglycosides, penicillins and diuretics are examples of drugs that fall into this group.

8: **Prescribing in the elderly**

Prescribing in the elderly and infirm carries an increased risk of adverse reactions. This is in part related to high tissue drug levels, polypharmacy and inappropriate timing of doses. Compliance may also be an issue in some cases.

Pharmacokinetics

Absorption

This is not substantially different in elderly people.

Distribution

Elderly people may have very low body weights and are thus susceptible to overdose. Furthermore, they tend to have a lower percentage of total body water but a higher proportion of fat compared to young adults. There is therefore a risk of accumulation of lipid-soluble drugs in more elderly patients.

Metabolism and excretion

The metabolism of some drugs is variable in older people relative to younger people. However, in general terms, liver mass and blood flow are decreased and so inactivation of drugs is slower. The metabolism of other drugs appears to be relatively unaffected by age (e.g. warfarin). The issue is further complicated by the fact that many elderly patients are taking several medications and this will obviously further affect drug metabolism.

Both glomerular filtration rate and tubular function are decreased in elderly people. Drugs that are excreted by the kidneys, such as gentamicin or lithium, may need to be prescribed in lower doses.

General issues

The earliest sign of adverse or toxic effects is likely to be a non-specific malaise. Mild confusion, weakness and an altered bowel and bladder habit are common. Of particular importance are non-steroidal anti-inflammatory drugs (NSAIDs) and diuretics. In the elderly, NSAIDs lead to increased bleeding tendency into the gastrointestinal tract. The morbidity and mortality of such bleeds are greater in this group. In patients on NSAID therapy who develop peptic ulceration, every effort should be made to stop the NSAID and substitute with an alternative drug. A proton-pump inhibitor is then the best treatment. In elderly patients who are likely to require long-term NSAID treatment, prophylactic use of a proton-pump inhibitor should be considered.

Diuretics and a resultant low volume state may manifest as postural hypotension which may lead to falls and reduced mobility. Electrolyte disturbances are also more frequent. Sedatives and anxiolytics can induce confusional states.

The principles of prescribing in the elderly and infirm depend upon validating certain questions: is the drug absolutely needed and do the benefits in the elderly patient outweigh the risks?

1 Is there any benefit in the tight control of certain physiological parameters (e.g. does the blood glucose have to be between 4 and 7 in a chair-bound 90-year-old or can it be allowed to drift up to 10 or 12 safely)?

2 Will the route of administration be safe and effective in hospital and then in the community? Consider that the patient may prefer liquid or syrup forms of the medication you are prescribing. Consider also that the elderly patient may need assistance in the physical act of taking medications, either because of poor vision or arthritis.

3 The dosage should be reduced as necessary (see above) and there should be increased vigilance for side-effects and symptoms of toxicity. Long-acting agents that can accumulate (such as glibenclamide) should be avoided.

4 Prescribing intervals should be well defined and fixed, such as 'after every main meal'. The dosage should avoid significant fluctuations in plasma levels.

5 Over-the-counter preparations may cause interactions.

Follow-up

Follow-up should also be considered:

1 Regular review of the patient's condition and his/her prescription should be made while in hospital, including plasma levels if needed.

2 It is useful to arrange an appointment with the GP at the time of discharge from hospital to allow a further assessment and to set up regular reviews. A *Dosette* box, district nurse supervision or even day hospital care may all be needed.

3 In situations where there is a high risk of problems, repeat prescriptions should be for short intervals only.

9: Conception, pregnancy and breast-feeding

Prescribing for women of childbearing age should be done with care. Many otherwise safe drugs can have effects on the fetus, while others affect fertility in men and women. The *BNF* Appendix 4 has a comprehensive list of medicines and advice on prescribing during pregnancy, while Appendix 5 covers breast-feeding.

In order to clarify your intentions when prescribing, it is useful to consider the following points.

The patient's intentions:

1 Is the woman already pregnant?

2 Is conception likely or sought in the near future?

The disease process:

1 Is it an emergency?

2 If not, does the process need treating?

3 Is there a significant benefit to the woman?

4 Is there an equally efficacious, less potentially harmful alternative?

The drug, conception and the fetus:

1 Can the harmful effects be quantified?

2 Can the harmful effects be reduced in any way?

3 Is any form of screening available to detect harm?

Treatment of the pregnant patient

In an emergency, the clinical priority is the woman but it is vital that adverse effects to the fetus be stated immediately to the patient and family if unavoidable. One such example would be antiplatelet drugs and thrombolysis for a large myocardial infarction during the first trimester. The benefits to the mother are great but there is a very high risk of placental separation and hence abortion.

Most teratogenic effects occur in the first trimester. Second and third trimester problems occur during further tissue development and reflect toxic effects. Drugs at term may affect the process of delivery, the neonate, or both.

Treatment of the patient trying to conceive or at risk of conceiving

Certain drugs are significantly teratogenic. If they are needed, the patient must be advised to take measures to avoid conception. If pregnancy does occur, specialist opinion should be sought immediately and the risks evaluated as above.

Some drugs are teratogenic but their effects can be attenuated with other drugs and the benefits to the mother and secondarily to the fetus are great (e.g. anticonvulsants). Neural tube defects are possible but the incidence can be reduced by using smaller doses of single drugs and by prophylactic use of folate supplements. The risks of a seizure during labour are serious.

Table 9.1 A list of some of the common drugs that should either be avoided or used with caution in breast-feeding mothers. This list is not comprehensive.

Drug	Advice	Reason
Aspirin	Avoid	Reye's syndrome Reduced platelet function
Beta-blockers	Caution	Very low levels but observe child carefully
Captopril	Avoid	Gets into breast milk
Ciprofloxacin	Avoid	High levels in breast milk
Steroids	Caution	Trace amounts found above 40 mg/day prednisolone
Enoxaparin	Avoid	No evidence but based on manufacturer's advice
Frusemide (furosemide)	Safe	Levels probably too low for any effect
Antipsychotics	Caution/avoid	Very low levels seen but may affect immature nervous system
Paracetamol	Safe	
OCP	Only when weaning or after 6 months	Affects lactation
Ibuprofen	Avoid/caution	Very low levels but manufacturers suggest avoidance
Levothyroxine (thyroxine)	Safe	No effects on neonatal thyroid function tests
Lithium	Avoid	High levels in breast milk

OCP, oral contraceptive pill.

Specific drug treatments

Warfarin and heparin

Warfarin is teratogenic. A woman with a recent history of thromboembolism or deep vein thrombosis is at risk of a further event during pregnancy, which may be fatal. While heparin is not teratogenic, it does carry a significant risk of bleeding. On balance, the risk of bleeding is acceptable as it is small and, with good surveillance and immediate therapy, dangers can be minimized. In general, patients needing anticoagulation who are or who are at risk of becoming pregnant should be offered heparin therapy. Low molecular weight heparin can be used (see Chapter 22).

Methotrexate

This is an example of a drug that may cause fetal abnormalities even after cessation. Contraception should be used by couples if either partner has been on the drug during the preceding 3 months.

Chemotherapy

Cytotoxic drug regimens, especially those containing alkylating agents, will affect fertility adversely and most are teratogenic. This is a complex area and counselling by a specialist clinician is essential.

Breast-feeding

For breast-feeding, the situation is less critical as alternative methods of feeding exist. Here the effects may be on maternal lactation (dopamine agonists) or, more often, passage of the drug or its active metabolites into breast milk with resultant effects on the child.

A list of common drugs at standard doses that may have effects when given to breast-feeding women is shown in Table 9.1.

10: **Surgical patients: the preoperative stage**

This chapter is conc erned with the preoperative work-up of patients. It discusses which drugs to continue until the day of surgery, how to prescribe 'premeds' and how to deal with common preoperative problems, and then goes on to discuss the sedation issues of various procedures. Finally, local anaesthetics are considered.

It is becoming increasingly common that patients for elective procedures will have been assessed at a pre-admission clinic. These are designed to ensure that the patient is in the best condition for any operation. A thorough clinical review of the patient and his/her medication is needed to identify problems or drug interactions that need to be addressed. It is also good practice to inform the GP of the likely operation date and arrange for any further assessments.

Concurrent medications

Usually, medications that the patient is taking preoperatively should be continued until the day of surgery and even given on the morning of surgery itself. Giving these medications with a sip of water (even in a patient who is nominally fasted) is safe and appropriate.

Cardiovascular drugs

Generally, these should all be given, even if the operation is in the morning. Calcium antagonists can have additive effects on myocardial depression with induction agents, so inform the anaesthetist and observe local policy.

If the patient is on ACE inhibitors or diuretics, make sure that he/she is adequately hydrated, otherwise rapid changes in blood pressure can be seen on induction of anaesthetic. If the fluid status is uncertain, consider whether a catheter or another form of fluid monitoring is required.

Respiratory drugs

Maintenance levels of inhaled steroids, bronchodilators and antihistamines should be continued. If the airways disease is 'brittle', a preoperative review using spirometry and, possibly, a course of steroids are indicated. The anaesthetist should be alerted to this.

Antidepressants

These should be taken. Lithium at high doses can impair renal function and lead to a range of problems so adequate hydration is important. Check levels before the procedure and closely monitor renal function afterwards.

Monoamine oxidase inhibitors (MAOIs) interact with certain agents used on induction and should be stopped

2 weeks prior to surgery. This should have been addressed in the out-patient clinic when the patient was booked for theatre, possibly with transfer to another drug. The anaesthetist, GP and psychiatrist may all need to be involved in this decision.

Antiplatelet agents

There is an increased risk of bleeding with antiplatelet agents (e.g. aspirin). For major operations or those with a high bleeding tendency (e.g. prostatectomy), aspirin should be stopped 1 week before the procedure. The risk of central nervous system (CNS) embolic damage or ischaemic heart disease (IHD) is small compared to possible poor haemostasis. The need for antiplatelet agents with other procedures, such as cardiac surgery or coronary artery stenting, may be higher.

Anticoagulation

This is a very important aspect of perioperative care. It is covered in detail in Chapter 22.

Steroids

A history of steroid intake within the previous 6 months should lead to the consideration of steroid supplementation in the perioperative period. Although patients may have been steroid independent for a number of weeks, they may have an impaired stress response to surgery and need to be covered for this (see Chapter 24).

Diabetic medications

See Chapter 40.

Oral contraceptive pill and hormone replacement therapy

Oestrogens increase the risk of thromboembolism and so patients on the oestrogen-only pill, combined pill or HRT should discontinue this 1 month preoperatively. They should be counselled about the need to use alternative forms of contraception. Patients taking the progesterone-only pill do not need to stop this.

In patients undergoing emergency surgery, adequate thromboembolism prophylaxis, employing both mechanical methods and heparin, should be used (see Chapter 22).

Anaesthesia and premedications

Although anaesthesia is a speciality in its own right, there are a number of aspects of which every doctor should be aware. These include premedications as patients are often given these before leaving the ward; sedation/hypnotics, as these are a part of many procedures (e.g. endoscopy); and the after effects of general anaesthetics and local anaesthesia.

Anaesthetics

Anaesthesia may be general, regional, local, or a mixture of these. Muscle relaxation may be necessary either to facilitate the surgery (such as a laparotomy or the need for a precarious position), as an aid to ventilation or because the risks of aspiration are significant enough to require a definitive airway.

Muscle relaxants used are depolarizing (e.g. suxamethonium) or non-depolarizing (e.g. vecuronium). If a patient has had a depolarizing drug will have experienced generalized muscle contractions at the point of induction and may complain of aches and pains on waking. This is normal. If the muscle relaxants have not worn off adequately or been fully reversed with a cholinesterase inhibitor (e.g. neostigmine 2.5 mg i.v.), the patient may have problems with respiration. Low tidal volumes and poor oxygenation may be seen. This should have been looked for and excluded before return to the ward.

Induction of anaesthesia can be through any route but is almost universally intravenous or by inhalation. The 'white stuff' used is propofol, which is a commonly used drug in this situation. Etomidate has a less cardiac depressant effect and is used in elderly or unstable patients. Thiopental (thiopentone) is a potent barbiturate which is also used as an induction agent. The exact drug used is decided by the anaesthetist on an individual basis. It is at the time of induction of anaesthesia that cardiovascular instability will most often show itself.

Anaesthesia can be maintained through a number of routes. Volatile agents are most commonly used in the UK to acheive this. There are a number of these: sevoflurane and isoflurane are common. They have a spectrum of side-effects. The most apparent of these is a hangover sensation and nausea.

Analgesia intraoperatively is likely to be a combination of opiates, NSAIDs and regional or local blocks. Postoperative pain relief depends very much on the type of procedure and the anaesthetist (see Chapter 13).

A range of fluids, including blood products, may be used or lost in theatre. These should all be documented in the anaesthetic record, prescription chart and fluid chart. This is often inefficiently carried out. It is good practice to list the intraoperative fluids used on the drug chart and fluid chart.

Premedication

These are drugs given close to the operation time, i.e. if the patient is very anxious (benzodiazepines), or to dry secretions (e.g. hyoscine) as part of total analgesia provision (oral *Brufen*). You might consider use of a bronchodilator as a premedication, antibiotics or increase in steroids. Although it is still done in many areas, avoid using deep intramuscular premedications. They are painful, have unpredictable absorption and better routes are often available. Clarify the need for this with your anaesthetist.

Specific issues commonly encountered in the immediate preoperative period

Anxiety

Reassurance is often all that is needed, but occasionally short-acting benzodiazepines (temazepam 10 mg orally, 45 min preoperatively) can be of help. Often it takes much longer to wake up fully after the operation. This may particularly be an issue in day care patients.

After a patient has had sedating medication, it is questionable whether they are able to understand information or to give informed consent, so ensure that all necessary paperwork has been completed first.

Hypertension

If the blood pressure is genuinely elevated, check to see how these values compare to normal for the patient. Have the normal antihypertensives been taken and time allowed for them to act? If pressure is still elevated, beta-blockers, alpha-blockers or nitrates can be used. Usually at this point it is wise to inform the anaesthetist, who can assess the anaesthetic risks of the case and postpone surgery if necessary. In the majority of general cases an elevated blood pressure will not matter greatly, but in some operations it is *vital* to have low controlled systolic pressures to aid in haemostasis (e.g. head and neck operations, neurosurgery and ear, nose and throat (ENT) surgery). In adrenal surgery, pressure should be well controlled with both alpha- and beta-blockade before theatre.

Nausea and vomiting

Known significant postoperative nausea and vomiting should be taken seriously. Metoclopramide is ineffective in opiate-induced nausea. Cyclizine 50 mg i.v. is first-line therapy. For severe symptoms, ondansetron 8 mg i.v. 30 min preoperatively and postoperatively is of benefit.

See Chapter 35.

Deranged clotting

See Chapter 22.

Labile blood glucose

This should really have been addressed much earlier. If glycaemic control has just become unstable (normal range HbA1c but very high BM value), then always check if anything else has happened. Occult myocardial infarction is often a cause for such a problem. If the patient is on insulin therapy and on a sliding scale, check the ranges in your sliding scale and the fluids given. A gentle adjustment is usually enough (see Chapter 40).

Sedation and hypnotics

There are a number of procedures, such as endoscopy, during which sedation may be desirable. There is a choice of different medications used for this, some of which are listed below.

Midazolam

This is a short-acting water-soluble benzodiazepine that provides sedation and amnesia but not anaesthesia. It has a shorter duration of action than diazepam. It can be given intravenously, usually starting with 2 mg initially then increasing after 1 min or by 1-mg increments until adequate sedation is achieved. It may cause respiratory depression and so oxygen saturations should be measured in these patients. There is considerable interpatient variability in sensitivity to these agents. However, the elderly and those with chronic obstructive airways disease (COAD) are particularly at risk.

Excessive doses of midazolam (or if the drug is given too fast) may cause respiratory depression or arrest. Its effects can be reversed with flumazenil 200 micrograms over 15 s, with further boluses of 100 micrograms every minute as required up to a maximum of 1 mg. Midazolam is not routinely reversed because flumazenil itself is not without risks. Apart from causing nausea, vomiting and agitation, it may rarely cause convulsions.

Opioids

These drugs may aid both sedation and analgesia in patients undergoing procedures such as reduction of dislocations or fracture manipulation.

Antimuscarinics

These drugs may be used in endoscopy or radiology, predominantly to reduce smooth muscle spasm. They may cause confusion, vomiting and bradycardia.

Local anaesthetics

Local anaesthetics cause reversible blockade of the conduction of impulses in nerves by blocking sodium channels in the nerve membrane. They can be used either as topical agents, for infiltration of wounds and skin sites, or for specific nerve blocks. Most local anaesthetics are in the form of a base combined to a hydrochloride.

There are a number of considerations when choosing a local anaesthetic agent.

1 *Time to onset of effect and the duration of action.* A long duration of action is not always desirable as this may delay patient mobilization or discharge. Lidocaine has a rapid onset of action and moderate duration of effect. By contrast, bupivacaine has a slower onset but a longer duration of action.

2 *Percentage solution of drug.* For example, lidocaine is available in 0.5, 1, 1.5 and 2% solutions for injection and up to 4% as a surface agent. A solution expressed as 1% contains 10 mg of drug in 1 mL. For wound infiltration, a low-percentage solution is desirable as this allows the drug to reach a wide area. By contrast, for specific nerve blockade, with a more targeted delivery of the anaesthetic, a higher percentage solution might be used.

3 *Presence or absence of adrenaline.* To increase the duration of action of local anaesthetics, vasoconstrictors, usually adrenaline 1 : 200 000, are sometimes included with the local anaesthetic. This reduces the rate at which the local anaesthetic is taken up into the circulation. This has the additional benefit of decreasing bleeding if infiltration is being used prior to a surgical procedure. Adrenaline-containing solutions should never be used for infiltration around end-arteries (e.g. penis, ring block of fingers or other areas with a terminal vascular supply) as the intense vasoconstriction may lead to severe ischaemia and necrosis. The maximum dose of adrenaline is 500 micrograms (1 : 200 000 adrenaline contains 5 micrograms/mL).

Topical local anaesthesia is useful for skin and mucous membranes. In general, cocaine, lidocaine and prilocaine are the most useful for this purpose. The onset of action is usually 5–10 min and lasts for up to 1 h.

Table 10.1 Local anaesthetics: preparations and recommended maximum dosages.

Available preparations (% solutions)	Available preparations with adrenaline (% solutions)	Available topical preparations	Maximum doses (with adrenaline)
Lidocaine			
0.5, 1, 2%	0.5, 1, 2%	Gel 1, 2%, ointments 4%, EMLA (with prilocaine)	3 mg/kg (7 mg/kg)
Bupivacaine			
0.125, 0.25, 0.5%	0.25, 0.5%	None	2 mg/kg (2 mg/kg)
Prilocaine			
1, 4%		EMLA (with lidocaine)	6 mg/kg (9 mg/kg)
Amethocaine			
0.2%	None	Ametop 4%	

EMLA cream (Eutectic Mixture of Local Anaesthetics; lidocaine and prilocaine) is used to provide topical anaesthesia and is especially useful in children but not neonates. It should be applied 1 h in advance and is commonly used prior to taking blood or the placing of intravenous cannulae. An occlusive dressing will stop it being rubbed off. *Ametop* is similar.

Maximum doses and toxicity

Maximum doses are given for each local anaesthetic in Table 10.1. However, this is only a guide and plasma levels will be higher if the area injected is more vascular (e.g. intercostal block). The addition of adrenaline reduces the peak concentration in blood, but the degree of this reduction again depends on the site of injection and the specific local anaesthetic agent.

Maximum plasma levels of local anaesthetics usually occur at around 30 min. Signs of toxicity include mild sedation and circumoral paraesthesia. At higher levels, convulsions, cardiovascular collapse and rhythm disturbances may be seen.

Local anaesthetics with or without opiates are used to give spinal and epidural anaesthesia (Table 10.1).

11: Intravenous fluids

The body compartments

Sixty per cent of an adult male is water, meaning that the 'average' 70-kg male comprises 42 L of water. This percentage is slightly lower for females, as they tend to have more body fat. Fifty-five per cent of body water resides within the intracellular fluid and 45% is in the extracellular fluid (ECF). The ECF can be found in plasma, interstitial fluid, transcellular water and water associated with bone.

Water moves across the cell membrane if there is a difference in osmolality between the sides. The number of particles determines osmolality, not their size:

$$Osmolality = 2(Na + K) + glucose + urea.$$

The normal osmolality of ECF is 280–295 mOsm/kg.

Effects of infusion of common intravenous fluids

5% Glucose

The glucose within the infusion is rapidly metabolized resulting in, effectively, an addition of water to the intravascular compartment. This fluid should only be used to replace mostly pure water loss. This rarely happens, although diabetes insipidus is one example where an almost isolated water deficit is seen. It should not be used in acute fluid resuscitation.

Dextrose saline

This comprises 4% glucose with 0.18% saline. It is useful as the basis for providing basal replacement as it has 30 mmol of sodium and chloride with the glucose being rapidly metabolized leaving water. Hyponatraemia may occur with overuse of dextrose saline.

0.9% Normal saline

This contains 150 mmol/L of sodium and potassium and matches the intracellular osmolality. Thus, normal saline tends to distribute throughout the extracellular space without any net movement of water into the cells.

Colloids

These include albumin, starches and gelatins. The capillary membrane is impermeable to colloid and so the solution remains within the intravascular compartment for longer. Most of these carry a high salt load and this must be considered when planning therapy.

Intravenous fluid replacement

There are three aspects to planning intravenous fluid administration:

1 basal requirements;
2 additional requirements; and
3 correction of deficit.

Basal requirements

Basal requirements for an adult are about 30–40 mL/kg/day water and approximately 2 mmol/kg sodium and 1 mmol/kg potassium. This is in health and takes into account losses in sweat, faeces and urine. The very presence of a patient in hospital suggests that basal replacement alone may not be adequate to keep pace with increased losses.

Additional requirements

One of the most common examples of a patient with additional requirements occurs in bowel obstruction, vomiting or in those with a high nasogastric output. Indeed, a patient with bowel obstruction can easily lose 3000 mL of fluid from his/her nasogastric tube. This fluid is rich in electrolytes, especially potassium, and a fluid regimen should include this in addition to basal requirements. Pyrexia produces greater water and salt loss (an extra 200–300 mL per increase in 1°C). High-output stomas can lead to losses in bicarbonate, potassium, chlorine, sodium, water and protein. Bleeding will cause a proportionate loss of everything.

A spot assessment of urinary biochemistry, including pH, may help to guide replacement.

Correction of deficit

Normal saline is an ideal first choice in the majority of situations. It will buy you time to assess the patient further and plan therapy. Colloids stay in the vascular space for longer and may be more appropriate after the initial stage. If there is significant bleeding, you should cross-match blood in order to get a blood transfusion available as soon as possible.

Assessment of fluid deficit is a clinical judgement which should take into account physical signs, including the moistness of mucous membranes, blood pressure, pulse rate, jugular venous pressure and urine output. Further information may be obtained from blood tests and assessing renal function and haematocrit. In special cases, total urine output of electrolytes may need to be measured.

If you suspect that a patient has a fluid deficit, then it is reasonable to institute intravenous fluids without special tests. Crystalloid 250–500 mL over 1 h will rarely cause significant harm even in a 'well-filled' patient.

Assessment of fluid status and monitoring of correction

Fluid requirements

If there is concern about the level of deficit or about fluid overload, then serious consideration should be given to a urinary catheter and possibly a central venous pressure (CVP) line. The pressure reading from a CVP line is a reflection of right atrial pressure, which is usually 3–8 cm water. The absolute value of the CVP reading is affected by a number of different variables, including right heart function, superior vena cava calibre, exact position of the tip, respiration and the infusion of other fluids along the central line. However, most of these factors tend to cause an over-estimation of the CVP and so a low reading tends to be significant. Generally, more significant than the actual CVP reading is the response of the pressure to infusion of a volume of crystalloid, such as 250 mL saline. If the patient is dehydrated, there is an initial rise in CVP, which rapidly returns to baseline as the patient vasodilates to accommodate the extra fluid. If the patient is adequately filled, the initial rise in CVP of 2–4 cm of water is sustained for around 15–30 min before slowly returning to normal. If the patient is overfilled or the myocardium is failing, the rise in CVP may exceed 4 cm of water and will not fall again.

The timing of the correction of fluid deficit is a matter of judgement. If the deficit is not severe, then it is reasonable to make it up over 48 h. However, if some other intervention is planned, it may need to be faster. One such example would be the patient who needs a laparotomy for peritonitis. He/she is likely to be dehydrated, but resuscitation is only a bridge towards minimizing the risks inherent in surgery for peritoneal lavage and treatment of the underlying cause. Fluid replacement must be as rapid and effective as can safely be achieved before peritonitis and sepsis supervene.

Alternatives to central lines include femoral lines. These can be used to measure central pressure trends but are more prone to changes in intra-abdominal pressure compared to an internal jugular or subclavian line.

When a steady state has been achieved, a daily weight chart gives the most useful reflection of fluid status.

General issues

One myth is that if patients can eat and drink, they will sort out their own fluid state. This may be true in health and for the walking wounded, but for a considerable number of in-patients this is not the case. It is easy to imagine a scared old lady in a busy accident and emergency department with tepid water in a plastic jug, just out of reach. She may be scared to drink as she is worried no-one will be able to take her to the toilet. Sadly, this happens every day. The ability to eat and drink does not equate to the intake of adequate food and fluid and does not allow relatively rapid correction of established losses.

Fluids should be prescribed with any additives clearly indicated and the rate to be given noted. It is good practice to prescribe a maximum of 24 h of fluid at any time. Hyperosmolar fluids can cause damage to veins and should only be given through large vessels or centrally.

Supplements

Maintenance of plasma potassium levels is important and this can be achieved using oral or intravenous supplementation. The quantity of potassium that may be given intravenously over 24 h depends on the type of access. Peripheral veins may be damaged by giving concentrated solutions and hence it is not recommended to give more than 40 mmol/L potassium and at not more than 30 mmol/h. These are maximum values and if there is a need to give more potassium than these amounts, then a central line is appropriate and a more thorough review of the case may be

Table 11.1 Composition of various intravenous fluids.

Solution	Na (mmol/L)	Cl (mmol/L)	K (mmol/L)	mOsm/L
Normal saline	150	150	0	300
Hartmann's	131	111	5	280
5% Dextrose	0	0	0	280
Dextrose saline	30	30	0	286
Gelofusine	154	125	0.4	465

Cl, chlorine; K, potassium; Na, sodium.

necessary. When given centrally, the concentration of potassium is less important as long as the maximum dose does not exceed 30 mmol/h, unless under exceptional circumstances.

Calcium supplements may be given as chloride and gluconate salt. Calcium chloride 10% carries 680 micromol/mL of free calcium ions. Calcium gluconate 10% has 220 micromol/mL of free ions. Both come as 10-mL ampoules and calcium chloride also comes as a minijet. Whichever you use for a specific indication, it is best to have a dedicated small volume bag of carrier fluid and give it at about 2–3 mmol over 5 min.

Magnesium replacement is dependent upon indication. It is poor practice to add this to a maintenance fluid bag and a dedicated syringe or small bag of fluid should be employed. The initial dose is 8 mmol over 20 min for rhythm disturbances and 72 mmol over 12–24 h is the usual replacement rate (Table 11.1).

Table 11.2 Venous catheters and infusion rates.

| Colour | Gauge | Maximum infusion rate | |
		(mL/min)	(L/h)
Blue	22	30	1.8
Pink	20	55	3.3
Green	18	80	4.8
Orange	14	270	16.2

All crystalloid fluids can be supplemented with more electrolytes and the addition should be clearly marked on the fluid bag and the drug chart. A person having fluid and electrolyte therapy should have regular biochemical checks of renal function and electrolytes to guide the therapy.

Venous catheters are classified by colour and gauge (Table 11.2).

12: **Nutrition**

Up to half of patients in hospital may show evidence of malnutrition as a result of their underlying disease or their social situation. Malnutrition may be compounded by the process of hospital admission and treatment such as surgery. Poor nutritional status is associated with a number of problems including poor wound healing, reduced muscle strength, unbalanced electrolyte compositions and dehydration. This has significant morbidity and mortality. The dietetic services in hospitals should be considered an integral part of the team and their advice sought early. Assessment of nutrition is not simple. Some of the methods are shown in Table 12.1.

There is no single test that reliably identifies the patient with malnutrition. Therefore, it is good practice to assess all patients coming into hospital. Patients who are at risk of malnutrition tend to be identified by the following risk factors:
1 recent weight loss, greater than 10% of body mass;
2 impaired dietary intake prior to admission (e.g. dysphagia because of oesophageal cancer);
3 future reduced intake likely (e.g. prolonged ventilation or nil by mouth);
4 vomiting and/or diarrhoea; and
5 increased nutritional requirements because of underlying disease (e.g. sepsis).

Perhaps the single most important issue in nutrition is that patients with a normal or near-normal gastrointestinal tract should be fed via the enteral route. A meta-analysis comparing early enteral feeding with parenteral nutrition has shown a reduction in septic complications from 35% to 18% [1].

In general terms, the process by which a patient is fed may be based on the following factors:
1 Able to take food via the oral route and normal (or near normal) gut function: oral diet possibly with diet supplements.
2 Unable to take food via the oral route (e.g. poor swallow post-cerebrovascular accident, CVA) and viable gut function: enteral nutrition using tube feeding.
3 Unable to take food via the oral route and lack of access to the enteral route or a non-functioning gut: parenteral nutrition.

Most patients' requirements are adequately met by 2000–2500 kcal per 24 h and approximately 1.5 g of protein per kilogram (or 7–14 g of nitrogen per 24 h). Giving more than the necessary energy requirement may result in hyperlipidaemia and hyperglycaemia.

Malnutrition in patients with normal gut and able to eat normally

These patients should be encouraged to eat. In this group of patients, it is important to check that they are indeed getting

Table 12.1 Methods of assessing nutritional status. Note that the examples may be affected by many factors other than nutrition.

Method	Example
Anthropomorphic measurement	Triceps skinfold thickness
Dynamometric measurement	Hand grip strength
Biochemical measurement	Serum albumin
Immunological measurement	Lymphocyte count

an adequate nutritional intake. Poorly fitting dentures, bad eyesight, inability to reach the food placed on a bedside table or a dislike of the food itself can all contribute to poor intake. It is useful to ask nursing staff to keep a chart of food intake (both food ordered and amount of each meal eaten). Favourite meals can be brought in by the family but there are reheating rules to be followed, so seek out local policy.

There is a large range of cartons of liquid supplements available. One of the most commonly used is *Ensure*, which has 251 kcal in 250 mL volume and contains 10.0 g protein, 8.4 g fat and 33.9 g carbohydrate with additional minerals and vitamins. It comes in a range of flavours and is also available in powder form. Juices, powder supplements and milk shakes have all been formulated.* Some can be frozen to make ice-slushy type drinks.

It is the policy of certain units to supplement routinely the calories in a standard hospital meal. This is especially true in elderly care wards. Snack packs are now available in NHS hospitals, which can be ordered at any time of the day. These are individualized food packets. The exact contents vary but include a selection of fruit, biscuits, crisps, yoghurt and sandwiches. This is designed as a snack and should not be used repeatedly in lieu of a meal. These do not need to be prescribed.

Malnutrition in patients with normal gut but unable to take an oral diet

Routes of access

Many patients have a relatively normally functioning gut but have an impaired ability to take in food. This may be because they have swallowing problems (e.g. stroke) or diminished consciousness (e.g. being ventilated on an intensive treatment unit, ITU). In such patients, enteral feeding via a nasogastric or nasojejunal tube, percutaneous gastrostomy or feeding jejunostomy is appropriate. Apart from simplicity and avoidance of venous line-associated morbidity, this approach has several advantages over parenteral nutrition. It helps to maintain the intestinal barrier function, bowel mass, bowel flora and reduces the risk of stress ulceration.

A wide-bore feeding tube is preferable

---

* The enteral supplements are listed in Appendix 7 of the *BNF*.

if nasogastric aspiration is likely to be required and poor absorption is anticipated. Fine-bore tubes are more comfortable for longer term use. Feeding is commenced at a slow rate (e.g. 50 mL/h) and this is increased as tolerated by the patient. Sometimes, gastric stasis may hinder enteral feeding and this manifests as abdominal distension, high-volume nasogastric aspirates or vomiting. In such circumstances, promotility agents such as erythromycin (250 mg b.d. orally) or metoclopramide (10 mg b.d. orally or i.v.) may be helpful.

For any surgery after which prolonged postoperative enteral feeding is anticipated, a feeding jejunostomy is often placed at the time of surgery. This has the advantage of being less irritant to the patient. Furthermore, after surgery the colon and stomach take the longest time to recover motility. The small bowel, by contrast, often recovers almost immediately. Many upper gastrointestinal surgeons also favour jejunostomies because they allow feeding distal to the site of anastomosis.

Composition of enteral feeds

There are a number of polymeric enteral feeds available, which normally contain 1 kcal/mL and around 5 g protein per 100 mL. The overwhelming majority of patients can be adequately managed using a polymeric diet. In a small number of patients (e.g. those with short gut syndrome or pancreatic insufficiency), intraluminal hydrolysis may be limited and an elemental diet may be preferable. The nitrogen source in these feeds is from free amino acids or oligopeptides and carbohydrate is supplied in the form of glucose polymers of less than 10 glucose molecules. If using a nasally placed tube, the position is normally checked by an X-ray prior to starting feeding.

There is a trend towards early aggressive enteral feeding in patients. In wellnourished patients in whom oral or enteral feeding is not anticipated within 7–10 days of surgery, consideration should be given to early parenteral nutrition (see below).

Malnutrition in patients with abnormal or inaccessible gut

These patients require total parenteral nutrition (TPN). Some of the issues associated with parenteral nutrition are considered below.

Routes of access

The intravenous supplements are high osmolality and should be given through a dedicated cannula in a large vein. Some can be given peripherally but thrombophlebitis and line failure commonly occur. If prolonged use is envisaged, central access is needed. This should be clearly labelled and preferably isolated from the other lines. Lines can be tunnelled so that the exit point through the skin is remote from the site of venepuncture to reduce line infection risks.

Composition of total parenteral nutrition

TPN bags are normally 2.5–3 L in volume. Thus, it is rarely necessary to give additional fluid supplementation to patients, unless there are exceptional additional losses (e.g. fistulae, high nasogastric tube losses). They usually contain around 2000 kcal, provided approximately equally by carbohydrate and lipid emulsions. They also contain electrolytes, trace minerals and vitamins. The hospital pharmacist may adjust the proportions of each of these to take account of the daily electrolyte results.

Morbidity associated with total parenteral nutrition

There is considerable morbidity associated with the central lines commonly used for TPN. These are immediate complications associated with insertion, including arterial puncture, haemothorax and pneumothorax. There are also delayed complications, including line-related sepsis and venous thrombosis. It is partly in response to this that interest has been reawakened in the use of fine-bore peripheral cannulae and other measures known to reduce cannula occlusion, such as GTN patches. A 15-cm ultrafine cannula placed at the antecubital fossa may last for a couple of weeks if looked after carefully.

There are also metabolic complications associated with TPN, including hyper- and hypoglycaemia. Insulin regimens may be needed at the same time. Abnormalities of plasma potassium, sodium, calcium and phosphate are also seen. Regular monitoring of electrolytes and liver function is essential. It is common to see deranged liver function (predominantly cholestatic in pattern) amongst patients on long-term TPN.

Giving drugs via enteral feeding tube route

It is not enough to just prescribe drugs to be administered via the nasogastric route or similar. Most tablet or capsule forms of drugs can be crushed and given via the tube. Drugs that are slow- or controlled-release preparations are unlikely to retain this quality as crushing often disrupts the delivery system. Naturally long-acting agents can be used normally.

Prescribe suspensions when possible and replace slow-release drugs with short-acting agents given at increased frequency and comparable replacement doses. This is bound to disrupt established pharmacokinetics and closer monitoring may be needed for clinical effects and therapeutic plasma levels.

Absorption of drugs will be affected by the feeding regimen. Some drugs require an acid or alkali medium to activate so gastric or jejunal delivery can have significant impact. Details of such drugs are beyond the scope of this book and once the treatment intentions are clear, a discussion with your local pharmacy to select the most suitable drugs in the relevant classes is advised.

Once normal feeding commences, previous medicines can be reintroduced with vigilance regarding effects and levels.

Reference

1 Moore FA, Feliciano DV, Andrassy RJ *et al.* Early enteral feeding, compared with parenteral, reduces post-operative septic complications: the results of a meta-analysis. *Ann Surg* 1992; **216**: 172–83.

13: **Analgesia: management of acute pain**

Pain is a common problem. It can be defined in a number of different ways and means different things to different people. The subjective pain a patient feels may be compounded by anxiety and fear and it is important that these aspects are addressed. A regimen that on paper looks ineffective may have been providing good control of symptoms in the community. While there may have been a large psychological component to this, persuading your patient will be difficult. Although the science is debatable, a pragmatic approach is warranted here unless there is harm in continuing with the patient's drugs.

It is often useful to ask patients to score their pain on an analogue scale of 0–10, with 0 representing no pain and 10 the worst pain they have ever felt. This is useful in assessing the response to analgesics.

The basic principles of analgesia are:
1 regular dosing;
2 minimum doses required for pain relief;
3 consider non-pharmacological methods of pain relief;
4 combination therapy; and
5 regular review of analgesic needs and efficacy.

Acute intervention to regain control is called rescue analgesia and provision should be made for this whenever treating a painful condition.

Types of analgesic drug

Simple (non-opiate) analgesia

Paracetamol

This is a very good analgesic and also has antipyretic properties. It has less anti-inflammatory activity compared to NSAIDs. It is particularly effective when prescribed as a regular medication. It is generally safe but should be used with caution in patients with liver impairment. It is a dangerous drug in overdose. The resultant severe liver damage may not manifest itself for several days. Doses of 500–1000 mg can be given with a maximum dosage of 4 g in 24 h.

Aspirin

This is an NSAID and is also both an analgesic and an antipyretic. It also has antiplatelet activity. Its mechanism of action is through cyclo-oxygenase inhibition.

NSAIDs

When an anti-inflammatory effect is particularly being sought, many clinicans would prefer an NSAID other than aspirin, as these other preparations are often better tolerated. They are very useful drugs for the treatment of pain and are being increasingly used in the perioperative period to reduce pain and

Table 13.1 The Oxford league table of analgesic efficacy. Numbers needed to treat are calculated for the proportion of patients with at least 50% pain relief over 4–6 h, compared with placebo in randomized double-blind single-dose studies in patients with moderate to severe pain. Drugs were oral, unless specified, and doses are milligrams.

Analgesic (mg)	Numbers needed to treat
Ibuprofen 800	1.6
Ketorolac 60 (i.m.)	1.8
Diclofenac 100	1.9
Paracetamol 1000 + codeine 60	2.2
Oxycodone IR 5 + paracetamol 500	2.2
Rofecoxib 50	2.3
Diclofenac 50	2.3
Ibuprofen 400	2.4
Aspirin 1200	2.4
Pethidine 100 (i.m.)	2.9
Morphine 10 (i.m.)	2.9
Ketorolac 30 (i.m.)	3.4
Paracetamol 1000	3.8
Paracetamol 650 + dextropropoxyphene (65 mg hydrochloride or 100 mg napsilate)	4.4
Tramadol 100	4.8
Codeine 60	16.7
Placebo	N/A

i.m., intramuscular; N/A, not applicable

analgesic requirements. Diclofenac and ketorolac are just two examples of NSAIDs that can be given by injection (intravenous or intramuscular). Avoid intramuscular NSAIDs as they are painful. Ibuprofen 800 mg taken orally provides the most efficient analgesia for the maximum number of patients, as reported in the Oxford analgesia ladder in Table 13.1.

COX-2 inhibitors

Selective inhibitors of cyclo-oxygenase 2 (COX-2) have recently been developed. These drugs are, in broad terms, similar in efficacy to NSAIDs and cause similar qualitative side-effects. However, the incidence of upper gastrointestinal irritation or ulceration is lower with COX-2 inhibitors (see below).

Risks with use of aspirin, NSAIDs and COX-2 inhibitors

Aspirin should not be used in children under the age of 12 years, because of its association with Reye's syndrome and, although this is more unusual in older children, should be used with caution in the 12–16-year age group. It can cause angio-oedema and urticaria and also has an important interaction with warfarin, increasing bleeding risk.

Upper gastrointestinal side-effects

Gastric irritation or ulceration has been reported for aspirin and the other NSAIDs. Probably around 1200 patients die in the UK each year from NSAID-related ulcer bleeding or perforation [1]. These drugs should be taken with food. Enteric formulations of aspirin are available which should cause less gastric irritation, but at the expense of a slower onset of action.

Arthrotec contains diclofenac and misoprostol (a prostaglandin analogue). The misoprostol provides gastric protection in elderly patients with no gastric symptoms who need NSAIDs on a regular basis. The dosage is 75–150 mg/day.

COX-2 inhibitors have slightly more restricted licensed indications for use, which differ for the various preparations now available, although these are constantly being changed. Of importance, COX-2 inhibitors are associated with a lower incidence of side-effects — although they are still contra-indicated in the presence of peptic ulceration. The National Institute for Clinical Excellence (NICE) has recommended against the routine use of COX-2 inhibitors in the treatment of osteoarthritis and rheumatoid arthritis. It has been suggested that COX-2 inhibitors should be reserved for those patients at high risk of gastrointestinal side-effects (previous history of ulcers, perforation or bleeding). COX-2 inhibitors should also be considered in older patients or in those who are taking other medications known to increase the risk of upper gastrointestinal ulceration. There is no merit in combining COX-2 inhibitors with aspirin.

The newer intravenous COX-2 inhibitors, such as *Paracoxib*, are marketed for use in acute pain and have a prolonged therapeutic window (up to 24 h).

Exacerbation of asthma

Asthmatics may suffer increased bronchospasm with the use of NSAIDs. However, this is an uncommon problem. Patients who have well-controlled asthma and have previously taken NSAIDs without problems should be unaffected. A deterioration in the peak expiratory flow rate (PEFR) should prompt consideration of stopping the NSAID. It is inadvisable to start an NSAID in a patient with poorly controlled (or an exacerbation of) asthma.

Renal impairment

NSAIDs should not be used in patients with renal impairment. They can dramatically worsen renal function. In hypertension and heart failure, the condition can be made worse by fluid retention.

Weak opioids

Dextropropoxyphene

This is a mild opioid with about half the potency of codeine. It is often used in combination therapies with drugs such as paracetamol. It is rapidly going out of favour.

Dihydrocodeine and codeine

These drugs have similar pharmacology. By themselves, they provide limited analgesia and should not be used as a rescue alternative. They are mostly used in combination with paracetamol or aspirin.

Strong opioids

These drugs are effective for the treatment of moderate to severe pain, especially that of visceral origin. Along with analgesia, euphoria and dependency can be seen. Respiratory depression can be fatal.

Morphine (and its more soluble cousin, diamorphine) remains the gold standard of therapy. Its versatility, reproducibility of action and ubiquitous availability have contributed to its widespread use. There are faster acting opioids , with shorter half-lives, less dependence on renal clearance and fewer side-effects. They are becoming more fashionable but still largely remain in the realms of specialist use, probably because of expense. Morphine can be given via any route. When used to control true continuous pain, there is little danger of addiction or tolerance. Respiratory depression is seen if excess opioids are given for the amount of pain experienced. There is no ceiling effect.

Constipation with morphine is severe, so laxatives can be used early. Liquid formulations of morphine are available for patients who have difficulty in swallowing. Intravenous preparations give high plasma levels rapidly. Initial doses should be given in 1-mg increments over 30 s until control is achieved.

Opioids can be given via the intramuscular route. In cases where there is hypoperfusion of muscle groups (e.g. hypovolaemia, cardiogenic shock), this route is unpredictable and should be avoided. It does have a role in the postoperative stable patient (see Postoperative analgesia below). Do not give intramuscular injections to suspected cases of myocardial infarction as thrombolysis can lead to a nasty intramuscular haematoma. Subcutaneous administration is possible and is used widely in the palliative care setting. Diamorphine is chosen as it is more soluble. Rectal preparations also exist.

Of the other opioids, pethidine has weaker effects but releases less histamine than morphine and so has a use when patients suffer from any form of atopy, including asthma symptoms. There is a theoretical benefit in pancreatitis or gallstone disease where there is less effect on the sphincter of Oddi. Pethidine is largely used intravenously or intramuscularly.

Fentanyl is a synthetic opioid which is 200 times more potent than morphine at the same dosage. It has a shorter duration of action but a very similar profile otherwise. It is used in surgical analgesia and the transdermal route is especially favoured in the palliative care setting. The patches come in 25-, 50-

and 75-microgram doses and this reflects the hourly release of active agent through the skin. They last for 72 h and can be combined to give the necessary quantity.

At very high doses of opiate analgesia, methadone can be considered. It is a very good analgesic and may significantly reduce the quantity of opiate needed.

Opiates can be reversed by naloxone, 200 micrograms given intravenously. Naloxone has a shorter half-life than morphine and so this dose may need to be repeated or given as an infusion.

The WHO analgesic ladder

The World Health Organization (WHO) advocates the use of a three-step analgesic ladder for the control of pain [2]. It ascends from mild pain at the bottom of the ladder to moderate to severe pain at the top of the ladder. At each level, the ladder suggests the consideration of adjunctive therapy. These therapies include pharmacological treatments, such as dexamethasone and betamethasone, which may relieve pain through an anti-inflammatory effect and through reduction in oedema. Adjunctive therapies also encompass non-pharmacological treatments, such as transcutaneous electrical nerve stimulation (TENS).

The WHO analgesic ladder is widely employed and regarded by many as the best approach to the management of pain from whatever aetiology.

Step one: mild pain (simple analgesics ± adjuvants)

Mild pain should be treated with simple analgesics. The NSAIDs are particularly effective for the treatment of pain with an inflammatory component, such as muscle and bone pain or strains. If NSAIDs are being prescribed for their anti-inflammatory properties, they sometimes require higher doses than would be needed for their analgesic properties alone.

Step two: mild to moderate pain (weak opioids ± paracetamol ± adjuvants)

Mild to moderate pain should be treated with weak opioids either alone or in conjunction with mild analgesics.

Step three: moderate to severe pain (strong opioids ± paracetamol ± adjuvants)

Moderate to severe pain should be treated with strong opioids such as morphine. These strong analgesics may be less effective in certain pain conditions, including neuropathic pain (see below).

Failure to control pain

A fundamental part of analgesia is the regular review of a patient's response to treatment. If the drug has not alleviated symptoms, then check that the patient's clinical condition is not deteriorating and check the patient's drug chart. It is not enough simply to have written a prescription for a patient, you also need to check that the patient has been requesting it (if it is written as a p.r.n. prescription) and whether it has been given.

Patient controlled analgesia

See Postoperative analgesia below.

Other sources of help

Many hospitals have specialized pain teams, which often include an anaesthetist. They are often an invaluable source of help and may advise on analgesia and other techniques, such as nerve blocks and epidurals.

Responses to specific painful conditions

There are a number of conditions that sometimes respond better to specific non-analgesic treatments. These are listed in Table 13.2.

Postoperative analgesia

The pharmacological agents used for postoperative analgesia are the same as for the management of any acute pain. Regional blocks and epidurals are also used in the immediate postoperative period. Good postoperative analgesia is vital to reduce the extent of complications, aid healing and promote recovery.

Pain can be helped with physical supports, such as a pillow across the abdomen when coughing after abdominal aortic aneurysm repair or a support trough after a knee replacement. Your ward physiotherapist will be able to help. Muscle spasm and anxiety should be attended to as needed. As with analgesia for any indication, it should be regularly given with drugs for breakthrough pain readily available. Drugs to act on the side-effects of the analgesics, such as antiemetics and opiate reversal agents, should be provided.

The oral route may not be as predictable in the immediate postoperative phase because of nausea or the type of procedure and so intravenous, intramuscular or regional blockade is preferred. Oral medications should be introduced soon after operation using combinations of simple agents, NSAIDs and opioids given regularly.

Algorithm for regular/intermittent intramuscular analgesia

All patients must have intravenous access kept open with a running flush and there must be opiate reversal agents available. There must be cardiovascular

Table 13.2 Specific diseases or syndromes associated with pain in which non-analgesic drugs should be first-line therapy.

Cause of pain	Specific drug
Angina pectoris	Glyceryl trinitrate
Neuralgia (postherpetic or trigeminal)	Carbamazepine, amitriptyline
Migraine (severe)	Ergotamine (use with care)
Dysmenorrhoea	Oral contraceptive pill, mefenamic acid
Mastalgia	Gamolenic acid (evening primrose oil), danazol
Phantom limb pain	Clonazepam

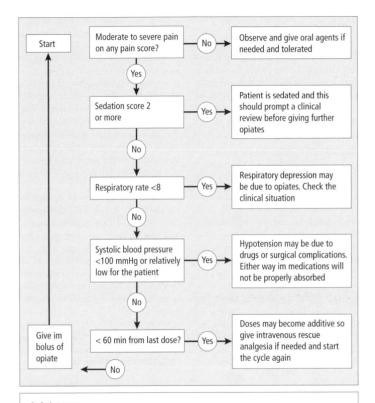

Sedation score
0 = awake and alert; 1 = slightly drowsy but rousable easily; 2 = quite drowsy but rousable;
3 = somnolent and difficult to rouse

Fig. 13.1 Algorithm for control of pain.

stability and the patient should not have a bleeding tendency. Use morphine whenever possible in a bolus dose of 7.5 mg for patients under 65 kg and 10 mg for those over 65 kg. The need for analgesia should be assessed at least every hour (Fig. 13.1).

Patient controlled (opioid) analgesia and epidurals

The principle is the same for these two modalities. A drug is administered via a regulated syringe driver. The amount of drug given is prescribed and boluses can be given either by the patient via a trigger or by an attendant (nurse/doctor). For patient controlled analgesia (PCA), any of the opiates can be used (commonly morphine or pethidine). For epidurals, local anaesthetic and opiate mixtures are used, although single agent versions are common.

Patient controlled analgesia

Patient controlled intravenous opiate analgesia is widely used in all branches of medicine to provide a consistent level of pain relief. Any opiate can be used although morphine still remains the agent of choice. Pethidine is more appropriate if histamine release could be a concern. The following should be undertaken in the patient requiring PCA.

1 Make 50 mg of morphine sulphate up to 50 mL saline or use a prediluted supply.

2 A dedicated specialized syringe driver is needed.

3 A constant background infusion rate may be set, although this is often not used.

4 The quantity for injection bolus is then set (usually 1 mg/1 mL morphine) and also its duration of infusion (usually immediately).

5 A lockout time is then defined during which no further drug can be given (typically 5 min). Some systems then require a maximum dose over 4 h to be set as a further safety feature against opiate toxicity.

There is usually a separate area on the drug chart for the prescribing of PCA. Some departments require every new syringe to be prescribed separately. While inconvenient in some respects, this does ensure a regular review.

For PCA to be successful, the patient must have had instructions preoperatively and have been able to understand them. There should be no physical limitation to activating the system (e.g. hemiplegia or severe rheumatoid hands). An intravenous loading dose of morphine should be given at the start of the process and provision made for a review of use a number of times a day. Naloxone should be readily available.

Do not prescribe regular opiates for use at the same time as a PCA (or opiate-containing epidural). Regular paracetamol and NSAIDs should be used when appropriate. Rescue analgesia should be available, which is best given as small increments of intravenous opiates until control is achieved once more. The reason for poor control can then be assessed (Table 13.3).

Check the venflon site but do not just flush through a used PCA line into the patient. Detach the line and then assess the patency of the venflon, the skin, presence of subcutaneous collections and, if in doubt, replace. This will allow you to test the rest of the kit at the same time.

Excess dosage may result in opiate toxicity. Assess the patient and reduce the opiate or stop it for a while. Stopping and reversing opiates fully results in pain that may be much more of a problem than the mild drowsiness. Clearly, if the patient is compromised, then you should resuscitate as usual, including the use of reversal agent (400 micrograms naloxone as a bolus followed by further doses or infusion if needed). When using pethidine PCA, doses above 1200 mg/day can

Table 13.3 Problem solving with patient controlled analgesia (PCA).

Problem	Cause	Actions
Not triggering the system enough	Patient control has failed	PCA may not be appropriate so reconsider its use
Triggering at high frequency	Significant opiate need	A full clinical review is needed Increase the background or bolus dose Add adjuvant drugs, e.g. regular paracetamol and NSAIDs
	Failure of apparatus or access	Check kit including venous access

NSAIDs, non-steroidal anti-inflammatory drugs.

lead to the accumulation of metabolites that can induce seizures.

Epidurals and patient controlled epidural analgesia

If your patient is to have a regional or epidural block, it is useful to know who is responsible for the prescription and, if there are any problems, who to call. You should familiarize yourself with the kit.

Epidurals (or patient controlled epidural analgesia, PCEA) involve a 24-G catheter inserted into the epidural space under aseptic technique. The active drugs are delivered to this via a biofilter (with pores small enough to stop some viruses). It is conventional for epidural tubing to be coloured yellow in the UK. Bupivacaine is a common local anaesthetic used. Combining with opiates does improve the quality of the block but can lead to respiratory depression. If opiates are to be used, fentanyl is relatively short acting and is a preferred agent, although diamorphine is also commonly chosen. If opiates are included in an epidural infusion, regular opiates should be avoided by other routes and great care taken to ensure close observations. In many cases, the pharmacy department will make up standard concentrations in syringes or bags.

> A typical epidural solution concentration:
>
> Bupivacaine 0.125% + fentanyl 4 micrograms/mL.
>
> In a 50-mL syringe this is equivalent to 62.5 mg of bupivacaine and 200 micrograms of fentanyl.

A thoracic epidural can start at a lower rate (4–6 mL/h) than a lumbar one (6–8 mL/h). If there is a patient controlled bolus, as in a PCEA, approximately 50–75% of the hourly dose is given as a bolus. This should be given over 2–5 min as the resistance in the fine catheter will not tolerate higher rates unless at very high pressures. A 30-min lockout should be used.

When the epidural is running, test the dermatomes for any analgesia (pain and temperature are carried together) and document your findings. If the block is poor but present, higher doses and greater volumes may be needed. This can be given as a rescue bolus followed by an increased hourly rate. If the epidural itself is not well placed the block may be patchy or non-existent. Unless you have been instructed in the care of this kind of kit, do not try to reinsert or manipulate it as you may do more harm. Seek assistance and if appropriately trained staff are unable to come, then cap off the lines, remove the catheter making sure the tip is seen and discard the syringe drivers for safety. Provide analgesia through conventional means.

Motor block can be seen with epidurals and this usually indicates a deep block. If you detect significant motor weakness or paralysis, stop the infusions and call for assistance. Possible causes are damage to the spine (unlikely) or a spinal block. A spinal anaesthetic is usually quite safe in experienced hands. As long as no further agent is given, it should wear off within a few hours. Try to sit the patient up to keep the block as low as possible. Problems occur if the block ascends and respiratory muscles are affected. Close observation and pulse oximetry are needed. A good marker for deep blocks or spinal blocks is a drop in blood pressure as peripheral vasodilatation occurs. It is important to closely monitor blood pressure, pulse, saturations and respiratory effort.

Ephedrine (predominantly alpha-agonist) given in 2–3-mg doses (it comes as 30 mg in 1 mL which should be diluted up to 10 mL of saline) can rescue profound hypotension caused by such vasodilatation. It will lead to a tachycardia as it is not selective. Give intravenous fluids also (250–500 mL of colloid over 30 min) if safe.

Respiratory depression can be seen with opiate toxicity and is dealt with in much the same way as in traditional PCA. The solution should be changed to a single agent (local anaesthetic only) and restarted once the patient has been resuscitated and after a full clinical review.

Continuous regional blocks

These have a similar sized (24-G) catheter placed in a nerve sheath or near a plexus. A solution of local anaesthetic is infused at a set rate. As yet there is no consensus on colours or identifying markers for these catheters or attachments so they should be clearly labelled at every port and connection.

References

1 Hawkey CJ. Non-steroidal anti-inflammatory drugs and peptic ulcers. *Br Med J* 1990; **300**: 278–84.
2 World Health Organization. Publication that described management of cancer pain. Geneva: WHO, 1996.

14: The acute surgical abdomen

This is a term that encompasses a range of surgical diagnoses including inflammation and/or infection, perforation, obstruction, infarction and haemorrhage. These conditions may affect a range of intra-abdominal organs. Some of the more common conditions are dealt with in more detail below.

General principles

Analgesia

As soon as a diagnosis has been achieved, analgesia should be commenced. The timing of analgesia is one of the controversies of surgical practice, with some practitioners maintaining that it interferes with the accurate assessment and monitoring of clinical signs. However, there is little evidence to support this in the literature [1]. Oral analgesia is often avoided in this group of patients, as many will be undergoing surgery.

Fluid resuscitation

Fluid balance must be optimized as far as reasonably possible, especially if surgery is being contemplated. This should include correction of dehydration and electrolyte disturbances, both of which are commonly seen in this patient group. Treatment should be instituted and monitored on the basis of clinical signs including pulse, blood pressure and urine output.

Antibiotics

These may be appropriate in certain cases and are considered in more detail below. In general terms, the acute abdomen may be managed surgically or non-surgically. The choice of antibiotic is determined by the site and type of pathology. The stomach and duodenum have low bacterial counts and perforation of these organs causes a peritonitis that is predominantly chemical in nature. Bacterial counts are also low in the small bowel. By contrast, large bowel perforations may cause considerable Gram-positive and Gram-negative bacterial contamination.

Acute appendicitis

The treatment of acute appendicitis is almost invariably by appendicectomy, with minimal delay. However, in patients in whom surgery is delayed for reasons of need for resuscitation or availability of theatre time, some surgeons advocate the use of broad-spectrum antibiotics such as cefuroxime 750 mg i.v. and metronidazole 500 mg t.d.s. i.v. However, most surgeons would agree that resolution of symptoms and signs on this antibiotic treatment should not prevent planned appendicectomy.

In all cases of appendicectomy, antibiotics should be given as a single pre-operative or perioperative dose as this reduces the incidence of postoperative wound infection [2]. A recent Cochrane review has supported this and suggested that the incidence of intra-abdominal infection may also be reduced [3]. In cases of perforated or gangrenous appendix at surgery, between 2 and 5 days of postoperative antibiotics should be given.

The treatment of uncomplicated appendicitis with antibiotics alone has been advocated [4]. This has not been widely adopted as appendicitis may progress to perforation. A relapse may also be seen in the medium term that will then require surgical intervention.

There are three notable exceptions where medical therapy should be preferred over surgery:

1 Medical facilities for appendicectomy are not available or are unsuitable.
2 Patient comorbidity mandates conservative treatment.
3 Appendix mass with localized signs.

In these instances, fluid resuscitation, analgesia and antibiotics (metronidazole 500 mg t.d.s. i.v. and a cephalosporin such as cefuroxime 750 mg t.d.s. i.v.) are commenced. This should be combined with regular clinical assessment and ultrasound if available. An associated abscess requires drainage and evidence of progressive increase in size of the mass, generalized peritonitis, persistent pyrexia and tachycardia may necessitate surgical intervention. Interval appendicectomy is usually performed some 2–3 months after the acute presentation. In older patients, this is usually preceded by a barium enema to rule out caecal carcinoma mimicking appendicitis.

An important differential diagnosis of appendicitis is pelvic inflammatory disease (PID). The gold standard for diagnosis is laparoscopy, although treatment is often based on a clinical diagnosis and vaginal swabs (which may be normal even in laparoscopically documented PID). The most common causative organisms in PID are *Chlamydia trachomatis* and *Neisseria gonorrhoea*, although other organisms are commonly involved. Inevitably, empirical treatment is often instituted with a quinolone orally and metronidazole 400 mg t.d.s. orally for 14 days. PID is associated with risks of tubal occlusion and infertility. Oral and rectally given metronidazole has very high bioavailability and is much cheaper than the intravenous route. In the acutely ill patient, especially if there is gastrointestinal upset, gut absorption is unpredictable and so the intravenous route is preferred.

Cholelithiasis and biliary colic

Gallstones are common, although in many patients they will cause no symptoms. Indeed, in autopsy reports from the UK, there is evidence that only 10% of stones have been treated by surgery [5]. Gallstones may be treated by dissolution therapy, commonly ursodeoxycholic acid or chenodeoxycholic acid. These drugs are suitable for those patients with a functioning gallbladder, radiolucent stones less than 2 cm in diameter and patients who are unfit for surgery. Patients should be advised to adopt a low-fat diet and they need to be monitored radiologically. These drugs have not been widely adopted, not least because the stones recur in around 25% of patients within 1 year of stopping drug treatment.

Colic is caused by sudden and complete obstruction of the cystic duct by a stone impacted in Hartmann's pouch. The pain is typically severe and usually lasts less than 12 h. If the duration of attack extends beyond this, then cholecystitis is a more likely diagnosis. Many cases can be safely managed at home by administration of opiate analgesia. Vomiting often accompanies the attack. If the patient fails to settle then hospital admission may be necessary.

Acute cholecystitis

The overwhelming majority of cases of cholecystitis are caused by gallstones or gallbladder sludge becoming impacted in the gallbladder neck and causing blockage of the cystic duct. This causes pressure within the gallbladder to increase and an inflammatory response is initiated. Bacterial infection with enteric organisms, most commonly *Escherichia coli*, *Enterococcus* and *Klebsiella* may occur. Such bacterial contamination occurs in about 20% of cases of cholecystitis.

The management of acute cholecystitis is a balance between conservative measures and operative intervention. It is appropriate to institute conservative measures in all patients presenting acutely and in the majority of cases the stone or sludge will fall back from the gallbladder neck. Such management includes nil by mouth, intravenous rehydration and analgesia. Analgesia might include morphine and an antiemetic. A single dose of 75 mg diclofenac i.m. has been shown to be beneficial in accelerating recovery from acute cholecystitis [6].

If the patient has systemic evidence of infection (temperature, raised white cell count) or is failing to settle, intravenous antibiotics should be started. This should usually be a second- or third-generation cephalosporin, such as cefuroxime 750 mg–1.5 g t.d.s. i.v., and metronidazole 500 mg t.d.s. i.v.

In some centres, conservative management is continued until symptoms settle and the patient is discharged with a view to interval cholecystectomy some 6–12 weeks later. However, not all patients will settle with conservative measures and urgent surgery will be mandated.

Complications of acute cholecystitis requiring urgent surgery

Around 10% of patients presenting with cholecystitis develop gangrene of the gallbladder. This is most common in men over the age of 50 years, with cardiovascular disease and a white cell count of over 17 000 leucocytes/mL [7]. This condition, or suspicion of it, requires emergency cholecystectomy. Gallbladder perforation presents with biliary peritonitis, although sometimes the perforation may be contained by adherent viscera and an empyema develops. After appropriate resuscitation, surgery is indicated.

Anaerobic infection of the gallbladder may also occur although this accounts for only around 1% of cases overall. It usually results from infection with clostridia or anaerobic streptococci, recognized by gas within the gallbladder wall, visible on plain X-ray or ultrasound. It can occur in the absence of gallstones. After appropriate resuscitation and broad-spectrum antibiotics, emergency surgery is usually performed as a high percentage proceed to perforation.

In patients unfit for surgery or very unwell, ultrasound-guided percutaneous drainage or surgical cholecystostomy are alternative measures to cholecystectomy.

Surgical intervention

Around 80–90% of patients with cholecystitis settle with conservative management. The issue of whether to opt for interval cholecystectomy or immediate surgery is contentious. However, there is evidence that those patients operated on within 72 h of the onset of symptoms have fewer complications and a lower conversion rate to open cholecystectomy than those patients operated on during the acute admission but after 72 h and those offered an interval cholecystectomy some 2–3 months after acute presentation [8]. This is said to be because during the acute phase of cholecystitis the oedema makes the dissection planes easier, but in surgery taken beyond this time, fibrosis has set in. However, there are further studies in direct contradiction to this, showing that conversion rates and morbidity are higher in patients operated on in the early (less than 3 days) phase of acute cholecystitis [9].

Ascending cholangitis

This classically presents with the Charcot's triad: epigastric pain, rigors and jaundice. It is always associated with a degree of biliary tract obstruction, with stones responsible in over 80% of cases. Relieving the obstruction is an essential part of management after initial medical therapy. This is most easily performed by endoscopic retrograde cholangiopancreatography (ERCP) and sphincterotomy but, if this fails, then percutaneous transhepatic drainage should be tried. Surgical drainage is a last resort.

Initial management, however, is medical and includes fluid resuscitation and antibiotics. The most common organisms involved are *E. coli*, *Enterococcus* and *Klebsiella*. An antibiotic regimen such as cefuroxime 1.5 g t.d.s i.v., metronidazole 500 mg t.d.s. i.v. is appropriate, with the addition of gentamicin in more ill patients. Such treatment is a temporary bridge to biliary tract decompression.

Acute pancreatitis

The treatment of uncomplicated pancreatitis is medical and essentially supportive in nature. The patient needs hospital admission, aggressive fluid resuscitation and catheterization to facilitate monitoring of urine output. Large amounts of fluid may be sequestered by the pancreas. Furthermore, the vomiting that often accompanies the condition may exacerbate the problem. A nasogastric tube is often beneficial. Oral intake may be recommended when pain and the associated ileus are settling. Early commencement of TPN should be considered.

Antibiotic use

The use of prophylactic antibiotics in pancreatitis is controversial. However, there is little evidence for their routine use in cases of mild pancreatitis, unless they are used to treat a specific infection

[10]. There are three trials pointing to the benefits of the use of antibiotics in severe pancreatitis with pancreatic necrosis. These have shown a reduction in septic complications, but no influence on mortality, possibly because the trials were underpowered [11–13]. However, a further trial showed a reduction in mortality with no effect on pancreatic sepsis [14]. Meta-analysis of these data has suggested a benefit both in terms of the reduction in septic complications and mortality with the use of antibiotics in acute severe pancreatitis [15].

The choice of antibiotic is unclear. Imipenem has been suggested on the basis of good penetration into pancreatic tissue, while cefuroxime prescribed early in the attack has been shown to reduce the incidence of infective complications and mortality. The duration of use remains unclear. Local complications of pancreatitis, including infected necrosis, pancreatic abscess and infected fluid collections, may require drainage by radiological or surgical means in addition to antibiotic treatment.

Platelet-activating factor antagonists

In patients with severe acute pancreatitis, there is some evidence that 3 days of treatment with a platelet-activating factor (PAF) antagonist reduces the severity of organ failure. However, more recent trials have thrown doubt on the effectiveness of this therapy and further studies are awaited.

Other drugs

A number of different agents have been tried in pancreatitis but without evidence of their efficacy. These include anticholinergics, glucagons and somatostatin. Gastric acid antisecretory agents are widely prescribed in pancreatitis, although direct evidence of their benefit is lacking. However, because the incidence of stress ulceration in these patients is known to be high, these seem to be reasonable therapy.

Chronic pancreatitis

Chronic pain is a major feature of chronic pancreatitis. If possible, nonsteroidal drugs should be tried as opiates may cause constipation and exacerbate abdominal pain. Fentanyl patches may be a useful alternative for patients poorly controlled with non-steroidals.

Pancreatic exocrine insufficiency manifesting as steatorrhoea is seen in a proportion of patients with chronic pancreatitis. These patients should be encouraged to reduce fat intake. Pancreatic supplementation (pancreatin) can be given. As these preparations are inactivated by stomach acid, they should be taken with food or, alternatively, a proton-pump inhibitor or H_2-receptor antagonist should be given.

Diverticulitis

Diverticulitis is defined as inflammation of colonic diverticula and pericolonic tissue by bacteria normally resident in the colon. The question of when to use antibiotics is determined by the clinical features; signs of severe inflammation or peritonitis should certainly prompt antibiotic use. In general terms, the treatment of diverticulitis is supportive and aims to prevent complications. Broad-spectrum antibiotics should be employed. The main causative organisms are aerobes, such as *E. coli*, *Proteus*, *Klebsiella* and enterococcus, and anaerobes, such as *Bacteroides*, *Clostridium* and *Bifidobacterium*. Many treatment regimens are based on metronidazole and a cephalosporin or gentamicin. These may be given intravenously if the patient requires in-patient care or orally if out-patient treatment is considered appropriate.

Many clinicians regard computerized tomography (CT) of the abdomen as the gold standard investigation in diverticulitis. This serves not only to confirm the diagnosis but also to assess whether there are any complications of diverticular disease, such as pericolic abscess, that may benefit from radiological drainage. This may accelerate recovery with conservative management.

Surgery is reserved for the complications of diverticulitis or in patients failing to settle or deteriorating with conservative management. Some authors advocate that elective surgery (usually sigmoid resection) should be undertaken in any patient with two documented episodes of diverticulitis.

Perforated peptic ulcer

When the diagnosis has been made, a nasogastric tube should be inserted to minimize intra-abdominal contamination. Analgesia and intravenous fluids are given. Antibiotics should be started: cefuroxime 750 mg t.d.s. i.v. and metronidazole 500 mg t.d.s. i.v. are commonly used. After resuscitation, most patients will be taken to theatre for oversewing of the peptic ulcer and suturing of an omental patch to the defect. At the time of surgery, these perforations have often sealed themselves; the critical aspect of surgery is the peritoneal lavage. Prompt use of a nasogastric tube and intravenous antibiotics also minimizes the intra-abdominal contamination. Many surgeons also prescribe ranitidine 50 mg t.d.s. i.v. immediately both for its ulcer healing actions and for reducing acid production and the 'chemical' peritonitis that characterizes perforated peptic ulcers.

After surgery, most would agree that patients need to be on either an H_2-blocker or a proton-pump inhibitor. The duration of this treatment depends on local policy, although some advocate lifelong treatment. As soon as reasonably possible, *Helicobacter pylori* should be sought and treated as necessary (see Chapter 36).

A proportion of patients are suitable for conservative management. This certainly includes the elderly patient with a 'silent' perforation-free gas under the diaphragm on erect chest X-ray without peritonitis. These patients should receive fluid resuscitation and intravenous antibiotics, such as cefuroxime 750 mg t.d.s. i.v. and metronidazole 500 mg t.d.s. i.v. Ranitidine 50 mg t.d.s. i.v. should also be commenced and a nasogastric tube passed. Some surgeons advocate the wider application of this non-surgical management to acute peptic ulcer perforation [16], although this has not been adopted widely. However, the issue of case selection makes such publications difficult to interpret. If the conservative approach is to be adopted, then regular clinical assessment is mandatory.

Peritonitis

Peritonitis is most commonly seen secondary to intra-abdominal disease such as perforated appendicitis, perforated diverticulitis, perforated peptic ulcers, trauma or perforated cancers. The principles of management of some of these conditions are covered above. Surgery (or, more accurately, peritoneal lavage) is commonly needed to prevent a downward spiral in the patient's condition. However, antibiotic therapy should be instituted as soon as the diagnosis of peritonitis has been made. This will probably need to be continued for several days postoperatively. The causative organisms are both anaerobes, such as *Bacteroides*, *Fusobacterium* and *Clostridium*, and aerobes, such as *E. coli*, *Klebsiella* and *Proteus*. A cephalosporin and metronidazole are commonly employed. The cephalosporin may be substituted by an aminoglycoside such as gentamicin. Gentamicin had fallen out of favour in recent years because of the risk of nephrotoxicity and the need to monitor serum levels. The evolution of a once daily dosage has resulted in a resurgence of its popularity.

In some centres, where the patient is very unwell or the degree of contamination is severe, monotherapy with a very broad-spectrum antibiotic, such as imipenem, is preferred. If antibiotics of such broad spectrum are used, there is a significant risk of candidal superinfections.

References

1 Attard AR, Corlett MJ, Kidner NJ, Leslie AP, Fraser IA. Safety of early pain relief for acute abdominal pain. *Br Med J* 1992; **305**: 554.

2 Krukowski ZH, Matheson NA. Ten year computerised audit of infection after abdominal surgery. *Br J Surg* 1988; **75**: 1023–33.

3 Andersen BR, Kallehave FL, Andersen HK. Antibiotics versus placebo for prevention of postoperative infection after appendicectomy. *Cochrane Database Syst Rev* 2001; **2**: CD001439.

4 Eriksson S, Granstrom L. Randomized controlled trial of appendicectomy versus antibiotic therapy for acute appendicitis. *Br J Surg* 1995; **82**: 166–9.

5 Godrey PJ, Bates T, Harrison M, King MB, Padley NR. Gall stones and mortality: a study of all gall stone related deaths in a single health district. *Gut* 1984; **25**: 1029.

6 Akriviadis EA, Hatzigavriel M, Kapnias D, Kirimlidids J, Markantas A, Garyfallos A. Treatment of biliary colic with diclofenac: a randomised, double-blind, placebo-controlled study. *Gastroenterology* 1997; **113**: 225–31.

7 Merriam LT, Kanaan SA, Dawes LG *et al*. Gangrenous cholecystitis: analysis of risk factors and experience with laparoscopic cholecystectomy. *Surgery* 1999; **126**: 680–5.

8 Eldar S, Eitan A, Bickel A *et al*. The impact of patient delay and physician delay on the outcome of laparoscopic cholecystectomy for acute cholecystitis. *Am J Surg* 1999; **178**: 303–7.

9 Pessaux P, Tuech JJ, Rouge C, Duplessis R, Cervi C, Arnaud JP.

Laparoscopic cholecystectomy in acute cholecystitis: a prospective comparative study in patients with acute vs. chronic cholecystitis. *Surg Endosc* 2000; **14**: 358–61.

10 Glazer G, Mann MV. United Kingdom Guidelines for the management of acute pancreatitis. *Gut* 1998; **42**: S1–13.

11 Pederzoli P, Bassi C, Vesentini S, Campedelli A. A randomised multicenter clinical trial of antibiotic prophylaxis of septic complications in acute necrotizing pancreatitis with imipenem. *Surg Gynecol Obstet* 1993; **176**: 480–3.

12 Delcenserie R, Yzet T, Ducroix JP. Prophylactic antibiotics in treatment of severe acute pancreatitis. *Pancreas* 1996; **13**: 198–201.

13 Nordback I, Sand J, Saaristo R, Paajanen H. Early treatment with antibiotics reduces the need for surgery in acute necrotizing pancreatitis: a single-center randomized study. *J Gastrointest Surg* 2001; **5**: 113–20.

14 Sainio V, Kemppainen E, Puolakkainen P *et al.* Early antibiotic treatment in acute necrotising pancreatitis: a prospective randomised trial. *Lancet* 1995; **346**: 663–7.

15 Golub R, Siddiqi F, Pohl D. Role of antibiotics in acute pancreatitis: a metanalysis. *J Gastrointest Surg* 1998; **2**: 496–503.

16 Crofts TJ, Park KG, Steele RJ, Chung SS, Li AK. A randomised trial of nonoperative treatment for perforated peptic ulcer. *N Engl J Med* 1989; **320**: 970–3.

15: **Vascular surgical issues: ischaemia (acute, chronic and prevention)**

Acute vascular ischaemia

Complete acute limb ischaemia results in extensive irreversible tissue necrosis within 6 h unless revascularization is performed. In those patients with incomplete acute ischaemia, medical therapy may result in limb salvage. If the limb is irreversibly ischaemic, amputation is required. This may have to be delayed depending on patient fitness or to allow demarcation if the level of amputation is uncertain. Otherwise, immediate amputation is required.

The two most important features of complete ischaemia requiring emergency treatment are paraesthesia and paralysis. Urgent referral to a vascular surgeon is required. Once a diagnosis of acute complete ischaemia has been made, the next important step is to define the cause for the ischaemia. About 60% result from thrombosis of a pre-existing area of atherosclerotic disease (plaque rupture). The majority of the remainder are attributable to embolus, most commonly from the left atrium in association with atrial fibrillation. Rarer causes, such as aneurysm, dissection and trauma, should be considered. The aetiology of the ischaemia has implications for its management.

Immediate management for complete and incomplete acute vascular occlusions

General resuscitation and optimization of medical status should, as always, be the goal. Stop all vasoconstricting agents. Patients should be given a bolus dose of 5000 units of unfractionated heparin followed by a further 1400 units/h (see Chapter 22), assuming no contra-indications apply. In particular, heparin is contra-indicated in aortic dissection or if there is a history of multiple trauma, head injury or actual or recent intracerebral bleed. Acute limb ischaemia is painful and analgesics should be prescribed. Opiates are probably best.

In cases of complete arterial occlusion, the patient should be taken to theatre for embolectomy or thrombectomy. Most surgeons would agree that thrombolysis is not an option. In cases of incomplete arterial occlusion, embolectomy or thrombectomy is rarely successful. These patients may benefit from thrombolysis, and angiography should be carried out if available. This will image the distal vessels and provide information about possible surgical reconstruction and the state of distal run off vessels, which is of particular interest if thrombolysis fails.

Thrombolysis is a specialist procedure in which streptokinase or recombinant tissue plasminogen activator is infused into the thrombus down a cannula placed into the clot or thrombus. It is a specialist procedure that should only be undertaken by appropriately trained staff in specialist units.

Prostacyclin analogues are sometimes used for the treatment of critical limb ischaemia. These drugs do not have a licence for this indication and should only be used with specialist advice as the resultant vasodilatation may cause severe hypotension.

Subsequent management

Patients with an embolic cause of acute limb ischaemia should restart heparin after surgery immediately or with a short delay of around 6 h (thought to reduce the risk of haematoma formation). Warfarin should be prescribed indefinitely, although some advocate giving heparin for 48 h before commencing warfarin to counter the theoretical initial hypercoagulable state (see Chapter 22).

Prevention of peripheral vascular disease

In the patient with intermittent claudication, the risk that he/she will progress to critical ischaemia requiring amputation is low (less than 1% per year). However, the symptoms of claudication are a marker for underlying atherosclerosis and the risk of death from coronary events and stroke in these individuals is high (of the order of 5–10% per year) [1].

Lifestyle factors

Smoking cessation is important. Patients who smoke heavily are approximately three times more likely to develop intermittent claudication, and peripheral artery disease is related to the amount and duration of smoking. Nicotine replacement in the form of patches, sprays and gums approximately doubles the rate of people stopping smoking.

Exercise is also important and increases claudication distance by around 150% in patients who are compliant with the regimes [2]. Patients should be encouraged to walk to a point close to the maximal level of pain for around 30 min at a time, at least three times a week and for at least 6 months.

Reduction in cholesterol

Patients should be encouraged to eat healthily, and reduce in particular the amount of saturated fat in their diet. Cardiovascular complications are reduced by about one-quarter in patients who have peripheral vascular disease and have their cholesterol reduced by one-quarter [3]. This appears to be independent of sex, age and baseline cholesterol level.

Antiplatelet and anticoagulant drugs

There is good evidence that aspirin (75–325 mg/day; mean duration of therapy 19 months) reduces the risk in at-risk patients of vascular occlusion or the need for a graft from 25% to 16% [4]. This is in addition to its proven benefits in reducing myocardial infarction and stroke. Patients at risk of peripheral vascular events should be offered aspirin 75 mg o.d. and should be counselled that this may not have any effect on symptoms or claudication distance but is given for prophylactic reasons.

While there is evidence that clopidogrel is marginally superior to aspirin in preventing vascular complications and death in patients with overt atherosclerotic disease, the number needed to treat for 1 year to prevent one event was 196. The substantially greater cost of treatment with clopidogrel compared to aspirin means that clopidogrel has not been widely adopted. It should be considered in those patients with peripheral arterial disease who cannot take aspirin.

There is no evidence to support the use of oral anticoagulants in the management of peripheral vascular disease.

Antihypertensive drugs

Patients with hypertension should be treated even though, in the short term, a reduction in blood pressure may worsen their symptoms. The choice of antihypertensive is probably between a low-dose thiazide diuretic or an ACE inhibitor. ACE inhibitors should be used with caution (monitoring of renal function) as there is a high incidence of renal artery stenosis in this group. A selective $beta_1$-blocker or a calcium antagonist would be second choice. There is a theoretical concern that $beta_1$-blockers may unmask claudication in previously asymptomatic patients or worsen the symptoms of peripheral vascular disease. While this has proven difficult to demonstrate in clinical trials, certainly $beta_1$-blockers are contra-indicated in patients with severe peripheral vascular disease. Carvedilol has some intrinsic sympathomimetic properties which may make it useful in this setting.

Diabetic medications

Up to 20% of patients with claudication may have non-insulin-dependent diabetes mellitus (NIDDM) and this should be sought at the time of presentation. Good glycaemic control reduces the microvascular complications of overweight people with diabetes and metformin reduces large vessel complications [5].

Peripheral vasodilators

Oxpentifylline, naftidrofuryl oxalate, cinnarizine and inositol nicotinate are licensed for peripheral vascular disease. They have been shown in small studies to produce small increases in pain-free walking, but these improvements are not dramatic and these drugs are therefore not widely used.

Raynaud's syndrome

This clinical syndrome has a number of aetiologies and is characterized by a classical three-colour change precipitated by cold. Lifestyle changes, especially stopping smoking, are vital. Some relief is obtained from using nifedipine 5 mg t.d.s. orally.

References

1 Burns P, Gough S, Bradbury AW. Management of peripheral arterial disease in primary care. *Br Med J* 2003; **326**: 584–8.

2 Leng GC, Fowler B, Ernst E. Exercise for intermittent claudication.

Cochrane Database Syst Rev 2000; **2**: CD000990.

3 MRC/BHF Heart Protection Study of cholesterol lowering with simvastatin in 20 536 high-risk individuals: a randomised placebo-controlled trial. *Lancet* 2002; **360**: 7–22.

4 Antiplatelet Trialists' Collaboration. Collaborative overview of randomised trials of antiplatelet therapy. II. Maintenance of vascular graft or arterial patency by antiplatelet therapy. *Br Med J* 1994; **308**: 159–68.

5 UK Prospective Diabetes Study (UKPDS) Group. Intensive blood-glucose control with sulphonylureas or insulin compared with conventional treatment and risk of complications in patients with type 2 diabetes (UKPDS 33). *Lancet* 1998; **352**: 837–53.

16: **Breast problems**

Endocrine therapies in breast cancer

Some breast cancers depend on oestrogen for their growth. Depriving tumours of this driving force is an established treatment for breast cancer. In postmenopausal women, androgens, mainly from the adrenals, are converted into oestrogens by the enzyme aromatase, which is present in a range of breast tissues, including about two-thirds of breast cancers.

Tamoxifen

Tamoxifen has a complex pharmacology and is metabolized to a number of different compounds that have different activities. However, its most important role lies in stopping the proliferation of breast cancer cells that express oestrogen receptors. Such tumours are described as being oestrogen receptor positive (ER positive) and can be identified by pathologists on the basis of core biopsy or excision specimens from tumours.

Tamoxifen also has partial oestrogen agonist activity in some other tissues. This translates into providing protection against osteoporosis in postmenopausal women. Less helpfully, tamoxifen also causes endometrial proliferation that results in a time- and dose-dependent increase in the risk of endometrial cancer [1]. Prompt investigation of patients with vaginal bleeding is required.

Patients on tamoxifen also have an increased risk of thromboembolism.

A recent Cochrane review of patients with early breast cancer (detectable cancer restricted to the breast and local lymph nodes) has assessed the benefits of tamoxifen. It concludes that looking at randomized trials of tamoxifen taken for variable durations of time, the risk of recurrence and death is reduced. In patients who are ER positive (or ER status unknown), the risk of recurrence is reduced by 34% and of death by 20%. By contrast, there is no clear evidence of benefit in patients whose tumours are classified as ER negative [2]. This review goes on to state that there is good evidence that 5 years of treatment is of greater benefit than 1–2 years. There is no evidence at present of a benefit with more than 5 years' treatment, as this would probably be associated with a higher incidence of adverse effects including endometrial cancer.

Aromatase inhibitors

These are a class of drugs that inhibit the synthesis of oestrogen from androgens in postmenopausal women. Further long-term data are required before the place of these drugs in relation to tamoxifen becomes clear. There is some evidence that anastrozole may be superior in ER-positive patients with early breast cancer in terms of disease-free survival and contralateral breast cancer. Anastrozole use was also associated with a lower incidence of endometrial cancer, stroke and thromboembolic events, although the rate of fractures was higher [3]. This class of drugs probably should, at present, be considered in patients at high risk of deep venous thrombosis, pulmonary embolus and endometrial cancer.

Breast pain

Breast pain is common. There are two broad categories of breast pain: cyclical and non-cyclical. By definition, patients with cyclical mastalgia are premenopausal and typically report that their symptoms are worst in the week before their period. They tend to complain of pain often associated with lumpiness and swelling in the breast. Patients with non-cyclical mastalgia tend to be older. The pain may come from the breast itself but also from other areas, such as the chest wall, incorrectly interpreted by the patient as being within the breast.

Treatment

Many patients with pain are worried that they have cancer. This is an extremely unusual presentation and patients should be reassured after clinical examination. Some centres advise patients to avoid certain dietary substances, including caffeine and chocolate, although the evidence of causation with these agents is unclear.

First-line therapy for cyclical breast pain is usually evening primrose oil (containing gamolenic acid), up to six or eight tablets per 24 h. It may take several weeks to see any benefit and a minimum of 3 months' treatment should be given. In patients still complaining of severe symptoms, it is reasonable to try either danazol (200 mg o.d. orally) or bromocriptine (2.5 mg b.d. orally). Neither drug should be given to patients on oral contraception and it is worth noting that many patients find that their cyclical pain improves in any case after switching to mechanical forms of contraception. The majority of patients should obtain relief after this algorithm of treatment. In those with persistent symptoms, there are other options, including tamoxifen and gonadotrophin-releasing hormone agonists, although these drugs are not currently licensed for these indications.

The true origin of pain in patients with non-cyclical breast pain needs to be elucidated as this determines treatment. In those patients with breast wall pain—often little more than costochondritis—analgesics, particularly NSAIDs, should be prescribed. Those with persistent pain may benefit from injection of the painful spot or trigger point with a combination of 1% lidocaine and 40 mg methylprednisolone. Patients should also be advised to wear a good supporting bra.

Breast infections

Breast infections are common. They may occur in the lactating or non-lactating state and are occasionally seen in neonates. They should be treated with antibiotics, the choice of which is determined by the type of infection. In cases that do not settle, intravenous antibiotics may be required. In such cases not settling with antibiotic treatment or those in which there is a solid mass that cannot be aspirated, one must consider whether there is an underlying breast cancer.

Lactating infection

For lactating breast and neonatal infections, the causative organisms are usually *Staphylococcus aureus* or *Staphylococcus epidermidis*. Treatment should be commenced with flucloxacillin (or erythromycin in those who are allergic to penicillin). The mother should be encouraged to continue to drain milk from the affected segment and this is most easily done by continuing to breast-feed.

A deep abscess in the breast should be excluded by ultrasound or attempted needle aspiration. If a deep abscess is demonstrated, repeated needle aspiration or incision and drainage may be necessary.

Non-lactating infection

The principles of treatment are the same as for lactating infection: antibiotic treatment and drainage of any associated abscess. In non-lactating breast infections, however, the causative organisms are slightly different and, in addition to *S. aureus* and *S. epidermidis*, include enterococci, anaerobic streptococci and bacteroides. Treatment should reflect this fact and might typically be co-amoxiclav orally or, in penicillin-allergic patients, erythromycin and metronidazole.

References

1 The American College of Obstetricians and Gynecologists. *Obstet Gynecol* 2000; **95**: 1C–3C.
2 Early Breast Cancer Triallist's Collaborative Group. *The Cochrane Library. Issue 1.* Oxford: Update Software, 2003.
3 ATAC Trialists Group. Anastrozole alone or in combination with tamoxifen versus tamoxifen alone for adjuvant treatment of postmenopausal women with early breast cancer: first results of the ATAC randomised trial. *Lancet* 2002; **359**: 2131–9.

17: **Urological problems: benign prostatic hypertrophy, incontinence and infections**

Benign prostatic hypertrophy

This may be treated either surgically or by trial of medical treatment. The mainstay of medical treatment is the use of selective alpha-adrenoceptor antagonists. These relax the smooth muscle of benign prostatic hypertrophy (BPH) and may give rise to an improvement in urinary symptoms. These drugs can cause hypotension, especially with the first dose and in those people on other antihypertensive drugs. They should be used with caution in patients with hepatic and renal impairment. The newer alpha-adrenoceptor drugs, such as tamsulosin and alfuzosin, produce fewer side-effects.

The 5-alpha reductase inhibitor finasteride has been shown to reduce the size of large prostates, although it takes several months to achieve this.

Urinary incontinence

Urinary incontinence can be considered under two headings: stress incontinence, where exertion increases pressure within the bladder and overcomes the incompetent sphincter mechanism; and urge urinary incontinence in which there are involuntary contractions of the bladder detrusor muscle. Patients with stress incontinence may benefit from general measures, including weight reduction and pelvic floor exercises. Those patients with residual symptoms may benefit from surgery.

Urge incontinence may also be improved by conservative measures, although many patients also derive benefit with antimuscarinic drugs. These drugs reduce the contractions of the unstable detrusor muscle and increase bladder capacity. The use of these drugs may be limited by their side-effects, particularly dry mouth, blurred vision and drowsiness. They are contra-indicated in patients with glaucoma, myasthenia gravis, urinary retention or outflow obstruction, severe ulcerative colitis or megacolon and bowel obstruction or atony. Tolterodine may have fewer side-effects than oxybutynin.

Urinary tract infection

This is classically defined as the presence of pure bacterial growth of greater than 10^5 colony forming units/mL. However, this is not an absolute rule and pure growth of a bacterium at a lower count in a symptomatic patient must be assumed to be significant.

Urinary tract infections are more common in women than men, although in men they are more frequently associated with an underlying abnormality of the renal tract. Urinary tract infections are also seen in children and renal scarring occurs in a number of these patients. Renal scarring may be associated with poor renal growth, early hypertension and renal failure.

Causative organisms and treatment

Escherichia coli of bowel origin is the most common causative organism, with *Staphylococcus saprophyticus* common in sexually active young females. Other organisms include *Proteus*, *Klebsiella* and *Streptococcus faecalis*. Patients who have been catheterized or have had some other type of instrumentation may have *Staphylococcus epidermidis* infection.

Urine should be taken prior to the start of treatment for culture. Empirical treatment can be started with trimethoprim 200 mg b.d. orally, nalidixic acid 1 g q.d.s. orally, nitrofurantoin 50 mg q.d.s. orally or amoxicillin 250 mg t.d.s. orally. Lower doses of these antibiotics may be required in children. Treatment should be for 1 week, although in women with an uncomplicated urine infection, 3 days of antibiotics may be adequate. Around 40–50% of *E. coli* are resistant to amoxicillin and are also increasingly resistant to trimethoprim. This re-emphasizes the need for a urine sample to be sent for culture prior to the instigation of therapy.

Investigation of urinary tract infections

Local policies vary on the need to investigate the underlying cause, if any, of the urinary tract infection. Although there is no convincing evidence to support this, many centres advocate the investigation of all first urinary tract infections in children and women with an ultrasound scan. Ultrasound provides good anatomical information without radiation exposure. Any abnormalities detected on ultrasound may direct subsequent investigations.

The investigation of urinary infections in men is more controversial. This group more commonly has abnormalities with an incompletely emptying bladder and stones being the most important factors. Many centres use intravenous urography (IVU) as their first investigation of choice as this should provide information about both abnormalities. However, there are risks associated with the use of such contrast media and there is a reasonable radiation dose. This approach has recently been challenged by others, including the suggestion that ultrasound and plain abdominal X-rays are as effective as IVU in the detection of pathology, although IVU may be important as a follow-up investigation in patients found to have an abnormality [1].

Prophylactic antibiotics

Local policies are again variable in this regard but many centres advocate prophylactic antibiotics in those patients with recurrent infections or evidence of renal scarring.

Pyelonephritis

Acute pyelonephritis can cause septicaemia. It should be treated aggressively and may require hospital admission. Treatment is normally with a broad-spectrum antibiotic such as cefuroxime 750 mg t.d.s. i.v. or ciprofloxacin 500 mg b.d. orally. Note that ciprofloxacin is as efficacious orally as it is intravenously. The former route is simpler and cheaper and should be preferred in all but occasional circumstances.

Reference

1 Andrews SJ, Brooks PT, Hanbury DC *et al*. Ultrasonography and abdominal radiography versus intravenous urography in investigation of urinary tract infection in men: prospective incident cohort study. *Br Med J* 2002; **324**: 454.

18: Deep vein thrombosis prophylaxis and the surgical patient

The need for deep vein thrombosis prophylaxis

The risk of death from pulmonary embolism (PE) has prompted the use of various methods to reduce the risk of deep vein thrombosis (DVT). Thirty per cent of patients over the age of 40 years undergoing major surgical operations develop DVTs if no prophylaxis is used [1]. This figure is even higher when one considers many forms of orthopaedic surgery or pelvic surgery. Nor is the risk restricted to patients undergoing surgery, with one study identifying as many as 20% of medical patients having DVTs after CVA or myocardial infarction (MI) [2].

The risk factors for venous thromboembolism are shown in Table 18.1.

Methods of prophylaxis

There are essentially three methods of combating DVT: early ambulation, mechanical methods and anticoagulation. Early ambulation of postoperative surgical patients and medical patients has become *de rigueur*, although some of this relates to financial issues and pressure on beds. The increasing use of day surgery has also contributed to shorter in-patient stays and early mobilization.

Graduated compression stockings are a simple form of mechanical prophylaxis. An alternative method is intermittent pneumatic compression which is preferred in some hospitals. Whether these two methods are synergistic or not remains controversial.

Anticoagulation usually involves heparin: either unfractionated (UF) or low molecular weight (LMW) heparin. Neither type of heparin, when used at prophylactic doses, requires monitoring with blood tests. UF heparin is usually prescribed as 5000 units b.d. or t.d.s. subcutaneously, while the dose of LMW heparin depends on the type of LMW heparin preferred. Warfarin has also been examined as a method of prophylaxis but is not commonly used.

Stratification of risk

Patients can be stratified into three levels of risk: high, medium or low (Table 18.2) [3]. The determination of the level of risk dictates the type of prophylaxis required. Low-risk patients should have graduated compression stockings, because there is little risk associated with their use, although they should not be used in people with peripheral vascular disease (Table 18.3).

Evidence for use of prophylaxis

There is evidence from randomized trials for the use of mechanical methods of prophylaxis in surgical patients,

Table 18.1 Risk factors for deep vein thrombosis (DVT).

Patient factors	Disease or procedure characteristics
Age over 40 years	Trauma or surgical procedure especially of lower limb
Severe obesity	Malignancy
Immobility	Heart failure
Pregnancy/puerperium	Recent MI
High-dose oestrogens	Paralysis of lower limb
Previous DVT or PE	Severe infection
Thrombophilia	Inflammatory bowel disease
Homocystinaemia	Nephrotic syndrome
	Polycythaemia
	Paraproteinaemia
	Behçet's disease
	Paroxysmal nocturnal haemoglobinuria

MI, myocardial infarction; PE, pulmonary embolism.

Table 18.2 Risk assessment of deep vein thrombosis (DVT).

Level of risk	Characteristics
Low	Patients under 40 years undergoing major surgery with no other risk factors
	Patients undergoing minor surgery with no other risk factors
	Patients with minor illness, history of DVT or PE, but no thrombophilia
Medium	Major surgery in patients over 40 years with one or more risk factors
	Major medical illness such as MI, chest infection, heart failure
	Major trauma
	Minor surgery, trauma or illness in patient with history of DVT, PE or thrombophilia
High	Fracture or major orthopaedic surgery on pelvis, hip or leg
	Major pelvic or abdominal surgery for cancer
	Major surgery, trauma or illness in patient with previous DVT, PE or thrombophilia
	Leg paralysis
	Critical leg ischaemia or major leg amputation

MI, myocardial infarction; PE, pulmonary embolism.

although the benefits are in reducing the incidence of DVT, with no clear evidence for a reduction in the incidence of PE. This may, in part, be a reflection of many of the studies in this field being underpowered to show a benefit in reducing PE. Furthermore, there is no clear evidence of benefit in the use of mechanical methods of prophylaxis in medical patients.

The benefits of heparin in surgical patients of medium risk and above and in patients with heart failure and chest infection are a little clearer [4]. LMW heparins are at least as effective as UF heparin for most forms of surgery and,

Table 18.3 Stratification of risk of developing deep vein thrombosis (DVT) and prophylaxis recommendations.

	Risk of proximal DVT (%)	Risk of PE (%)	Recommended prophylaxis
Low	0.4	<0.2	Early ambulation and compression stockings
Medium	2–4	0.5	Early ambulation, compression stockings and/or intermittent pneumatic compression, anticoagulation
High	10–20	1–5	Early ambulation, compression stockings and/or intermittent pneumatic compression, anticoagulation

PE, pulmonary embolism.

in general surgical patients, LMW heparins may be associated with less risk of bleeding [5].

Orthopaedic patients are at particularly high risk of DVT and PE. A recent meta-analysis concluded that LMW heparins are probably more effective in the prevention of DVT compared to UF heparin or warfarin for this group [6]. The risks of minor bleeding were reduced in the LMW heparin group but the study lacked sufficient power to comment on the risk of a major bleed.

References

1 Kock A, Bouges S, Ziegler S, Dinkel H, Daures JP, Victor N. Low molecular weight heparin and unfractionated heparin in thrombosis prophylaxis after major surgical intervention: update of previous meta-analyses. *Br J Surg* 1997; **84**: 750–9.

2 Nicolaides AN. ABC of vascular diseases. *Br Med J* 1991; **303**: 1323–6.

3 Verstraete M. Prophylaxis of venous thromboembolism. *Br Med J* 1997; **314**: 123–5.

4 Cook DJ, Guyatt GH, Laupacis A, Sackett DL, Goldberg RJ. Clinical recommendations for the use of antithrombotic agents. *Chest* 1995; **108**: 227–30S.

5 Palmer AJ, Schramm W, Kirchhof B, Bergemann R. Low molecular weight heparin and unfractionated heparin for prevention of thromboembolism in general surgery: a meta-analysis of randomised trials. *Haemostasis* 1997; **27**: 65–74.

6 Palmer AJ, Koppenhagen K, Kirchof B, Weber U, Bergemann R. Efficacy and safety of low molecular weight heparin, unfractionated heparin and warfarin for thrombo-embolism prophylaxis in orthopaedic surgery: a meta-analysis of randomised clinical trials. *Haemostasis* 1997; **27**: 75–84.

19: **Antibiotic prophylaxis**

This chapter considers prophylactic antibiotics in three groups of surgical patients. The first is those patients in whom the aim is predominantly prevention of wound infection associated with surgery. In the second, prophylactic antibiotics are given to patients with valvular or heart lesions in order to prevent endocarditis. The final group includes patients who have undergone splenectomy and require prophylaxis against future risks of sepsis. In each of these groups, patients with clinical evidence of infection preoperatively should receive appropriate treatment as part of the preoperative work-up.

Prevention of wound and infective complications associated with surgery

The risk of infection following a surgical procedure depends primarily on the type of surgery being carried out. This can be divided into three types: clean, clean–contaminated and contaminated (Table 19.1). The use of prophylactic antibiotics broadly follows these different categories. Clean operations may not require any antibiotic prophylaxis, although some surgeons prefer to give a single dose of prophylactic antibiotics on induction to cover the introduction of skin commensals. For clean–contaminated and contaminated procedures, antibiotic choice is determined by the site of surgery and the bacterial colonization of the field of operation.

The choice of antibiotic should be bactericidal rather than bacteriostatic. Peak antibiotic levels must be achieved at the time of operation itself and so the first dose should be given either a couple of hours prior to the operation or on induction of anaesthesia.

The duration of treatment, as a general rule, is three doses for clean–contaminated surgery (one on induction and two postoperative doses), while for contaminated surgery the duration of treatment is typically 5 days.

Prophylactic antibiotics form only part of the measures against infective complications. Hydration, nutrition and the treatment of intercurrent but distant infections should be addressed. Those patients considered at risk of methicillin-resistant *Staphylococcus aureus* (MRSA) should be swabbed if possible prior to surgery and isolation procedures and alternative antibiotic prophylaxis should be instituted in accordance with local policy. This is especially so if prostheses are planned.

General surgery

See Table 19.2.

Orthopaedics

Joint replacement

For elective total hip replacement, the

Table 19.1 Classification of types of surgery by characteristic features and postoperative risk of clinical infection.

Type of operation	Features	Risk of infection (%)
Clean	No mucosal breach No infection or inflammation	1–2
Clean–contaminated	Mucosal breach but no contamination	10
Contaminated	Preoperative infection Intraoperative contamination by breach of viscus	30

Table 19.2 Type of procedure, common causative bacteria in postoperative infection and suggested antibiotic prophylaxis.

Type of operation	Type of organisms	Suggested antibiotic regimen
Lower gastrointestinal surgery	Gram-positive and Gram-negative organisms, anaerobes	Cephalosporin and metronidazole *or* gentamicin and metronidazole *or* augmentin
Upper gastrointestinal surgery	Gram-positive and Gram-negative organisms	Gentamicin *or* cephalosporin
Appendicectomy	Gram-positive and Gram-negative organisms, anaerobes	Metronidazole suppository alone *or* cephalosporin and metronidazole
Biliary surgery	Gram-positive and Gram-negative organisms	Cephalosporin
Hernia surgery (with mesh) and surgery involving implants (e.g. vascular grafts, joint replacements, see below)	Skin commensals	Penicillin and flucloxacillin if mesh or implant is to be used or patient is high risk
Amputations or major trauma	Skin commensals, contaminants but also at risk of *Clostridia* (gas gangrene and tetanus)	Benzylpenicillin *or* metronidazole

incidence of wound infection is approximately 1%. Risk factors for any infective complications include diabetes mellitus, rheumatoid disease, malignancy, long operation duration and repeat surgery. Although the majority of infections present within the first 6 months, many present more than 2 years after surgery. Despite this, the organisms responsible almost always originate from the time of surgery. Blood-borne spread from a distant focus of infection or following procedures such as urinary catheterization is rare. The most common bacteria causing infection are *Staphylococcus epidermidis* and *S. aureus*, with MRSA becoming increasingly important [1].

Trauma

Wound infection rates following the surgical repair of bone fractures are higher than those seen after elective procedures—perhaps of the order of 3%. This probably reflects the poorer physical state of the patient and of the tissues surrounding the fracture. Bacterial organisms responsible for such infections are similar to those listed above for joint replacement.

The risk of wound infection following open fractures is substantially higher. Contamination is usually present preoperatively and soft tissue damage may be substantial. There may also be problems with skin or tissue coverage of the wound. Check the tetanus status of your patient in such a case. If he/she has not been immunized within the previous 10 years, this should be carried out.

General measures to prevent infection

There is good evidence that antibiotic prophylaxis for elective procedures in orthopaedics decreases wound infection rates. A total reduction of 76% in wound infection rates compared to those receiving no treatment or placebo has been shown in a recent systematic review [1].

A range of antibiotic regimens were examined and generally all seemed similarly effective in reducing wound infection rates. The duration of antibiotics ranged from a single dose at induction to 2 weeks. However, there are few data to support treatment beyond 24 h. There are similar data attesting to the usefulness of antibiotics in closed fractures. The choice of antibiotic prophylaxis prior to surgery for elective orthopaedics or closed fractures is usually a first- or second-generation cephalosporin (e.g. cefazolin or cefuroxime) or a penicillinase-resistant penicillin such as flucloxacillin. The choice of antibiotics for the patient known to have MRSA colonization or infection includes vancomycin and teicoplanin. However, the routine use of these antibiotics may undermine their usefulness in treating active MRSA infection through encouraging the emergence of more highly resistant pathogens. The use of these glycopeptides as routine is not therefore justified but may be appropriate in the individual patient with MRSA or in units with established MRSA problems.

In cases of open fracture, debridement and copious irrigation with saline or antiseptic are crucially important. Most surgeons would also advocate the use of antibiotics, although the few trials that exist in this area are poor in design and inevitably include a heterogeneous patient/fracture group. However, it is generally believed that antibiotics should be given, starting as soon as possible after the injury. This usually comprises a cephalosporin, often supplemented with either gentamicin or metronidazole. The duration of treatment is again unclear, although there is little firm evidence of benefit of treatment beyond

24h. Any subsequent evidence of sepsis, either local or systemic, should provoke the acquisition of swabs and blood cultures to enable the specific treatment of infection with a tailored antibiotic regimen.

Valvular heart disease

Patients with heart valve lesions, prosthetic valves, septal defects and patent ductus are at risk of endocarditis. They should therefore receive prophylactic antibiotic when undergoing dental procedures (dental extractions, scaling and surgery) or many forms of surgery [2]. These are summarized in Table 19.3.

Post-splenectomy prophylaxis

Splenectomy is performed for a range of indications including trauma. Splenic macrophages have a filtering and phagocytic role in removing bacteria and parasitized red blood cells from the blood. Loss of the spleen or functional hyposplenism leads to an increased risk of serious infections, particularly from encapsulated bacteria such as *Streptococcus pneumoniae*, *Haemophilus influenzae* type b and *Neisseria meningitidis*. Patients are also at risk from other infections, particularly malaria and those associated with animal bites. Sepsis from pneumococcal infection can have a high mortality rate. Asplenic patients require prophylaxis as outlined below [3].

Pneumococcal immunization

Patients should be given the pneumococcal vaccine 2 weeks before elective splenectomy. If not practicable, the patient should be immunized before leaving hospital or within 2 weeks. Reimmunization is required every 5–10 years. *Pneumovax* is given as 0.5mL subcutaneously. It should not be given in pregnancy or during breast-feeding.

Haemophilus influenzae type b immunization

Most children receive this vaccine in childhood and many adult patients will have acquired immunity through natural exposure. Patients not previously immunized should receive this. The issue of whether patients require reimmunization is unclear.

Meningococcal immunization

Protection with the current vaccine is short lived and covers groups A and C (B is most common in the UK). Therefore, routine post-splenectomy immunization is not recommended, unless there are specific indications such as travel abroad to areas where groups A and C are prevalent.

Influenza immunization

This is recommended yearly for those patients with immunosuppression caused either by disease or treatment. It may be of benefit for asplenic patients.

Antibiotics

Life-long antibiotics are recommended for all post-splenectomy patients. Oral phenoxymethylpenicillin 500mg b.d. is

Table 19.3 Type of procedure and antibiotic recommendations for patients at increased risk of endocarditis.

Procedure	Scenario	Antibiotic choice
Adult dentistry; under no anaesthetic or local anaesthetic only, no special risk	No penicillin allergy and no penicillin in previous month	Schedule A (Schedule B if penicillin allergic or penicillin taken in previous month)
Adult dentistry; under no anaesthetic or local anaesthesia only	Previously had endocarditis No penicillin allergy and no penicillin in previous month	Schedule C (Schedule D if penicillin allergic or penicillin taken in previous month)
Adult dentistry; under general anaesthesia, no special risk	No penicillin allergy and no penicillin in previous month	Schedule C (Schedule D if penicillin allergic or penicillin taken in previous month)
Adult dentistry; under general anaesthesia, special risk	Prosthetic valve or previously had endocarditis	Schedule E
Upper respiratory tract procedures		As for dentistry procedures
Genitourinary procedure	No urine infection	Schedule E (if urine is infected this also requires treatment)
Gastrointestinal, obstetric and gynaecological procedures	Only required for those who previously had endocarditis or prosthetic valve	Schedule E

Schedule A: amoxicillin 3 g orally 1 h before procedure.
Schedule B: clindamycin 600 mg orally 1 h before procedure.
Schedule C: amoxicillin 1 g i.v. at induction, then amoxicillin 500 mg orally 6 h later *or* amoxicillin 3 g orally 4 h before induction, then oral amoxicillin as soon as possible after the procedure.
Schedule D: vancomycin 1 g i.v. over at least 100 min, then gentamicin 120 mg i.v. at induction or 15 min before procedure *or* clindamycin 300 mg i.v. over at least 10 min at induction or 15 min before procedure, then clindamycin 150 mg orally or i.v. 6 h later.
Schedule E: amoxicillin 1 g i.v. and gentamicin 120 mg i.v. at induction, then amoxicillin 500 mg orally 6 h later.

recommended for adults, with lesser doses for children (250 mg b.d. for ages 6–12 years and 125 mg b.d. for age 5 years and under). In children in whom *H. influenzae* cover is required, amoxicillin may be used instead. However, even this does not cover *H. influenzae* re-liably. Patients allergic to penicillin should use erythromycin instead.

All patients should be warned that if signs of infection (fevers, rigors) develop, even if they are taking their prophylaxis correctly, they should present immediately to their doctor.

References

1 NINSS Partnership. *Surveillance of Surgical Site Infection in English Hospitals, 1997–99*. London: Public Health Laboratory Service, 2000.

2 Littler WA, McGowan DA, Shanson DC. Changes in recommendations about amoxycillin prophylaxis for prevention of endocarditis. Working Party of the British Society for Antimicrobial Chemotherapy. *Lancet* 1997; **350**: 1100.

3 Guidelines for the prevention and treatment of infection in patients with an absent or dysfunctional spleen. Working Party of the British Committee for Standards in Haematology. Clinical Haematology Task Force. *Br Med J* 1996; **312**: 430–4.

20: **Bowel preparation**

The clearing of the bowel (especially the colon) of faeces is an essential part of preparation of a patient for some forms of surgery, flexible sigmoidoscopy, colonoscopy and radiological investigations such as barium enema. A clean colon makes endoscopy easier and reduces patient discomfort. It makes radiological investigations easier to interpret as there is less faecal residue and reduced artefact.

General measures

Many hospitals have set policies on bowel preparation. However, some general guidelines are given below.

Laxatives

Patients being given oral laxatives should be asked to refrain from eating high-residue foods for 24–48 h prior to the procedure. While taking the oral laxatives listed in Table 20.1, they should be advised to drink plenty of water, although this is less important for those taking polyethylene glycol.

Oral laxatives work as osmotic agents that draw water into the gut lumen. They are universally contra-indicated in patients with bowel obstruction, perforation, megacolon, toxic colitis and ileus. There are a number of different preparations listed in Table 20.1 along with further drug-specific contra-indications

and cautions. Some may be used in children and manufacturers' instructions should be consulted for dosages where appropriate.

Enemas

Phosphates and sodium citrate may be given rectally either as a suppository or as an enema for bowel preparation. The use of this route of administration is variable between hospitals. The evidence for efficacy is reviewed below.

Before colonoscopy

Bowel preparation makes passage of the scope to the caecum easier and reduces patient discomfort [1]. A meta-analysis of eight randomized controlled trials comparing polyethylene glycol and sodium phosphate in patients undergoing colonoscopy has recently been published [2]. The endoscopist, who was blind to treatment, rated the preparation as acceptable more often in those patients taking sodium sulphate. Furthermore, 19% of those taking polyethylene glycol failed to complete the preparation, significantly more than those taking sodium phosphate.

A further study, comparing polyethylene glycol and magnesium oxide/citric acid/picosulphate in patients undergoing colonoscopy or barium enema showed that bowel preparation was similar. Finally, sodium phosphate has been

Table 20.1 Oral laxatives for bowel preparation.

Details of preparation	Timing of drug administration	Additional contra-indications
Sodium phosphate (Fleet Phospho-soda)		
45 mL bottles diluted with 120 mL water	For morning procedure: one bottle 8 a.m., one bottle 8 p.m. day before For afternoon procedure: one bottle 8 p.m. day before, one bottle 8 a.m. day of procedure	Congestive heart failure, renal failure, active inflammatory bowel disease. Not licensed for under 15-year-olds
Magnesium carbonate/citric acid (Citramag)		
Sachets, reconstituted with 200 mL hot water	Day before procedure: one sachet at 8 a.m., second sachet 6–8 h later	Severe renal failure. Not licensed for under 5-year-olds
Magnesium oxide/citric acid/sodium picosulphate (Picolax)		
Sachets, reconstituted initially to 30 mL then 5 min later to 150 mL	Day before procedure: one sachet in morning before 8 a.m., second sachet 6–8 h later	Severe renal failure, congestive cardiac failure. Not licensed for under 1-year-olds
Polyethylene glycol (Klean-Prep)		
Sachets, reconstituted in 1000 mL water	All four sachets within 4–6 h or until rectal effluent is clear. Two sachets may be taken day before procedure and two on morning of procedure	Use with caution if impaired gag reflex, gastro-oesophageal reflux or ulcerative colitis. Not licensed for children

shown to give superior preparation to magnesium oxide/citric acid/picosulphate in a trial involving 103 patients. There was no difference in tolerability of the preparation from the patients' perspective [3].

Before flexible sigmoidoscopy

This is a more limited endoscopic investigation compared to colonoscopy which aims to reach the splenic flexure. For this reason, many clinicians use enemas only as bowel preparation. These enemas are often administered in the hospital on the day of the examination. However, a recent study has shown that while many patients refuse to self-administer enemas at home, principally through a fear of not doing so correctly, amongst those who do, preparation is comparable and may be more acceptable to the patient, when compared to those patients receiving a hospital enema [4].

The issue of whether rectal compared to oral preparations give better bowel

Table 20.2 Guidelines for the use of bowel preparation (local practice may vary considerably from this).

Never
Bowel obstruction

Rarely
Small bowel resection
Strictureplasty
Upper gastrointestinal surgery
Colonic resection without anastomosis (e.g. Hartmann's and APR)
Formation of colostomy or ileostomy

Usually
Right hemicolectomy
Subtotal colectomy
Ileorectal anastomosis

Almost always
Anterior resection
Sigmoid colectomy
Left hemicolectomy
Anal sphincter repair
Anal reconstructive procedures

preparation remains controversial with conflicting results in the literature [5,6]. In summary, the data for optimal bowel preparation for flexible sigmoidoscopy are conflicting and local policy should be followed.

Before radiological investigation

Magnesium oxide/citric acid/picosulphate has been shown in two studies to give superior preparation compared to magnesium carbonate/citric acid [7] and polyethylene glycol [8]. Furthermore, polyethylene glycol caused more bloating and nausea. In a further study comparing magnesium oxide/citric acid/picosulphate to sodium phosphate, there was no difference in the quality of bowel preparation, although *Picolax* caused less nausea and vomiting [9].

Before surgery

Rationale behind bowel preparation

The rationale behind bowel preparation prior to surgical intervention includes reducing the bacterial load of the bowel, facilitating handling and palpation of the bowel, reducing wound and peritoneal contamination, reducing the chance of spillage and eliminating the proximal stool column, which some believe may disrupt the anastomosis. The question of which patients need full bowel preparation is contentious. Some surgeons do not use bowel preparation at all for elective cases, with seemingly low rates of complications [10].

Most surgeons use bowel preparation for all cases likely to involve colonic or rectal resection and primary anastomosis of large bowel to large bowel (Table 20.2). Many surgeons also advocate bowel preparation for cases in which the immediate postoperative passage of stool is potentially harmful to the patient, such as anal sphincter repair and anorectal reconstructive procedures. For operations involving small bowel resection and anastomosis only, most surgeons do not use formal bowel preparation but advocate 24–48h of low-residue or clear fluids prior to surgery.

In cases of elective right hemicolectomy and subtotal colectomy with primary anastomosis, most would also advocate bowel preparation although this is not universal. Some argue that, in these cases, small bowel is anastomosed to large bowel, no proximal stool column is present and primary anastomosis is safe. There is some indirect evidence to support this from the obstructed cases in which bowel preparation is contra-indicated and in which segmental colonic resection with on-table lavage was compared with subtotal colectomy without any form of bowel preparation [11].

Despite the widespread use of bowel preparation before colorectal surgery, there is little evidence for its benefit. There are only four randomized controlled trials comparing bowel preparation vs. no preparation and none shows a significant benefit for bowel preparation in terms of reducing wound infection, intra-abdominal wound infection and anastomotic leak [12]. However, each of these studies is probably underpowered.

References

1 Kim WH, Cho YJ, Park JY, Min PK, Kang JK, Park IS. Factors affecting insertion time and patient discomfort during colonoscopy. *Gastrointest Endosc* 2000; **52**: 600–5.

2 Hsu C-WL, Imperiale TF. Meta-analysis and cost comparison of polyethylene glycol lavage versus sodium phosphate for colonoscopy preparation. *Gastrointest Endosc* 1998; **48**: 276–82.

3 Yoshioka K, Connolly AB, Ogunbiyi OA, Hasegawa H, Morton DG, Keighley MR. Randomized trial of oral sodium phosphate compared with oral sodium picosulphate (Picolax) for elective colorectal

surgery and colonoscopy. *Dig Surg* 2000; **17**: 66–70.

4 Lund JN, Buckley D, Bennett D *et al.* A randomised trial of hospital versus home administered enemas for flexible sigmoidoscopy. *Br Med J* 1998; **317**: 1201.

5 Atkin WS, Hart A, Edwards R *et al.* Single blind, randomised trial of efficacy and acceptability of oral Picolax versus self administered phosphate enema in bowel preparation for flexible sigmoidoscopy screening. *Br Med J* 2000; **320**: 1504–8.

6 Bini EJ, Unger JS, Rieber JM, Rosenberg J, Trujillo K, Weinshel EH. Prospective, randomized, single-blind comparison of two preparations for screening flexible sigmoidoscopy. *Gastrointest Endosc* 2000; **52**: 218–22.

7 Chakraverty S, Hughes T, Keir MJ, Hall JR, Rawlinson. J. Preparation of the colon for double-contrast barium enema: comparison of Picolax, Picolax with cleansing enema and Citramag (2 sachets): a randomized prospective trial. *Clin Radiol* 1994; **49**: 566–9.

8 Hawkins S, Bezuidenhout P, Shorvon P, Hine A. Barium enema preparation: a study of a low-residue diet, 'Picolax' and 'Kleen-Prep'. *Australas Radiol* 1996; **40**: 235–9.

9 Macleod AJ, Duncan KA, Pearson RH, Bleakney RR. A comparison of Fleet Phospho-soda with Picolax in the preparation of the colon for double contrast barium enema. *Clin Radiol* 1998; **53**: 612–4.

10 Duthie GS, Foster ME, Price-Thomas JM, Leaper DJ. Bowel preparation or not for elective col-

orectal surgery. *J R Coll Surg Edinb* 1990; **35**: 169–71.

11 SCOTIA Study Group. Single-stage treatment for malignant left-sided colonic obstruction: a prospective randomized clinical trial comparing subtotal colectomy with segmental resection following intraoperative irrigation. Subtotal colectomy versus on-table irrigation and anastomosis. *Br J Surg* 1995; **82**: 1622–7.

12 Zmora O, Pikarsky AJ, Wexner SD. Bowel preparation for colorectal surgery. *Dis Colon Rectum* 2001; **44**: 1537–49.

21: **Wounds and abscesses, including dressings**

The management of wounds and selection of dressings is a complex subject, hindered in no small part by the fact that little evidence exists for many of the general principles of management or the selection of one type of dressing over another. It is worth seeking the advice of experienced nurses or, where available, wound care teams.

Wounds heal in two main ways: primary intention and secondary intention.

Primary intention

Wounds that heal by primary intention have their edges opposed and secured by sutures, clips, *Steri-strips* or tissue glues. These wounds do not normally require complex management. A simple occlusive dressing provides mechanical protection, protection from secondary infection and should be non-adherent for easy and pain-free removal.

A second important component of the management of such wounds is the removal of sutures. The operation note will specify the suture material used for closing the skin (Table 21.1). Absorbable sutures do not have to be removed. As a general but not infallible rule, absorbable sutures are clear and are often subcuticular (no visible external suture).

The timing of non-absorbable suture or clip removal is again variable. As a general rule, sutures on the head and neck should be removed after 3–7 days, chest and abdomen after 7–14 days and lower extremity wounds after 10–14 days.

Secondary intention

Wounds healing by secondary intention are open. They fill with granulation tissue and then contraction. Such wounds may be classified into a number of different types as shown in Table 21.2.

Types of dressing

Hydrocolloids (e.g. *Comfeel, Granuflex, Tegasorb*)

These dressings normally comprise an absorbent layer on a vapour impermeable film or foam. Their impermeability promotes autolysis and aids rehydration and moisture retention. They are usually self-adherent. They do not need to be changed daily but can be left in place for up to 1 week.

Hydrogels (e.g. *Intrasite, Granugel, Sterigel*)

These dressings are commonly supplied as an amorphous dressing that takes up the shape of the wound and can be moulded into the wound cavity. They often need to be covered with a non-adherent dressing or hydrocolloid. These dressings have a very high water content and increase hydration of the wound, thus promoting autolysis. They have some capacity for absorption of exudates. These dressings often need to be changed daily, at least initially. However, *Intrasite* must be left in place for up to 3 days and *Granugel*, which contains a hydrocolloid component in addition to hydrogel, may be left for up to 7 days.

Alginates (e.g. *Kaltostat, Sorbsan*)

These are prepared from calcium and sodium salts of alginic acid, a polymer prepared from seaweed. They are highly absorbent and are useful in leg ulcers with high exudates and also have haemostatic properties. These properties also make them excellent for packing abscess

cavities after surgical drainage. They are not appropriate for dry ulcers or wounds. The gelling characteristics of these dressing vary and those dressings that gel substantially may require moistening with saline to facilitate removal. The dressings may be left for over 24 h.

Foam dressings (e.g. *Allevyn, Lyofoam*)

Different foam dressings within this category may differ substantially. In particular, they differ in their absorptive capacity. Some of these dressings (e.g. *Allevyn*) are useful for moderately exudating wounds. Often, these types of dressing are used only as secondary dressings.

Vapour-permeable films and membranes

These allow the passage of water vapour and oxygen but not water or micro-organisms. They may allow inspection of the wound without dressing removal. They are useful in providing a moist environment for wound healing. However, they may not allow water vapour loss fast enough to prevent fluid accumulation under the dressing. This may cause skin wrinkling and dressing dis-

Table 21.1 Examples and properties of commonly used suture types.

Chemical nature	Examples
Absorbable	
Polyglactin	Vicryl
Polydioxanone	PDS
Non-absorbable	
Polyamide (nylon)	Ethilon
Polypropylene	Prolene
Silk	

Table 21.2 Type of wound and factors in selection of dressing.

Type of wound	Role of dressing
Hard, black, necrotic	Moisture rehydration or retention
Yellow, slough (rehydrated necrotic tissue)	Moisture retention or rehydration if dry or fluid absorption if wet
Green or red, exuding and granulating	Fluid absorption, thermal insulation
Pink, dry, with low exudate	Moisture rehydration or retention, thermal insulation and low adherence

ruption with entry of bacteria. They are less suitable for wounds with large amounts of exudates. They are often used as secondary dressings over alginates or gels.

Low-adherence dressings and wound contact materials

There are a number of different dressing types within this category.

Tulle or paraffin gauze dressings (e.g. *Jelonet*)

Tulle or paraffin gauze dressings comprise cotton or viscose fibres impregnated with yellow or white soft paraffin to prevent the fibres from sticking. However, the paraffin content reduces the ability of these dressings to absorb exudates. Medicated tulle dressings are also available and these may be impregnated with such compounds as sodium fusidate and chlorhexidine. There is no evidence of benefit of the antibacterial component of these dressings.

Povidone-iodine fabric dressings

These are knitted viscose dressings with povidone-iodine incorporated in a hydrophilic polyethylene glycol basis. Diffusion of iodine into the wound is facilitated, although this is probably rapidly deactivated by wound exudates. There is systemic absorption of iodine from these types of dressing.

Special situations

Cavity wounds

Any abscess or pus should be drained.

Traditionally, such wounds were packed with ribbon gauze, sometimes soaked in proflavine. Such gauze may be very difficult or painful to remove and the antibacterial properties of proflavine are not established.

Alginates (such as *Sorbsan* and *Kaltostat*) are probably the dressings of choice as they are capable of absorbing 15–20 times their weight in exudates. They are easily removed with saline. Hydrocolloid dressings may also be useful. They help with autolysis and are easy to remove.

Superficial burns

Place burnt area under cool running water for 10–20 min and give analgesia and reassurance. Non-adherent occlusive dressings are often helpful in this situation. Hydrocolloid dressings and vapour-permeable films and dressings may also be helpful.

Silver sulphadiazine cream is often used as a topical agent for superficial burns and may be helpful in reducing the bacterial load of the burn. It is sometimes helpful to cover the hands or feet afflicted by burns with a clear plastic bag. This allows physiotherapy and easy observation and monitoring of the wounds.

Leg ulcers

Non-adhesive occlusive dressings are often most useful. Typically, a hydrocolloid or hydrogel may be selected for a drier wound with little exudate. By contrast, an alginate may be preferable for an ulcer with a larger amount of exudate.

22: Anticoagulation

Unfractionated heparin

Heparin enhances the interaction between antithrombin III and thrombin and the factors involved in the intrinsic clotting cascade. It thus inhibits the action of thrombin in converting fibrinogen to fibrin and inhibits fibrin-induced platelet aggregation. Standard or unfractionated (UF) heparin has an average molecular weight of 15 000 and exerts its action on clotting through all of the above mechanisms. If intravenous UF heparin is to be used, it is usual to give this as follows:

1 5000 units UF heparin i.v. immediately;

2 25 000 units UF heparin made up to 50 mL with normal saline, to start running at 1400 units/h i.v. (2.8 mL/h); and

3 UF heparin, when used therapeutically, must be monitored by measuring the activated partial thromboplastin time (APTT). This should be 1.5–2.5 times control. This should be measured 6 h after commencement of therapy, and the rate of heparin infusion should be adjusted appropriately. APTT should be rechecked every 24 h or 6 h after changing the rate of heparin infusion, whichever is the sooner.

Fractionated heparin

Low molecular weight (LMW) heparin has an average molecular weight of only 5000 and has a greater capacity to potentiate the inhibition of factor Xa than it does to increase the inhibition of thrombin. The amount of heparin used depends on the patient's weight and the exact type of LMW heparin being used. For example, dalteparin is used at 200 units/kg subcutaneously for DVT or PE, and need be given only once a day as a one-off subcutaneous injection, up to a maximum of 18 000 units/day.

The use of LMW heparin does not require the measurement of APTT. It can be administered as a single daily dose and this has meant that many patients with uncomplicated DVT, for example, can be treated without admission to hospital. Most regions have adequate hospital based but community run anticoagulation policies.

Adverse effects of heparin

Bleeding

This is the most common adverse effect of heparin. In the case of UF heparin, if the APTT is above three times control, then the patient has an eightfold higher risk of bleeding. Usually, there is little need to do anything other than stop or reduce the infusion of UF heparin. LMW heparins do not usually cause as great a bleeding problem as UF heparin as the former has less action on platelet function.

However, it is possible to reverse

heparin (either UF or LMW) with protamine. This is given by slow intravenous injection and, as an approximate guide, 1 mg protamine reverses the effects of 80–100 units of heparin. If the heparin was given more than 15 min previously, then relatively less protamine is required, as the heparin is rapidly excreted. The maximum dose that should be given is 50 mg; if used in excess, protamine itself has an anticoagulant effect.

Thrombocytopenia

This is seen in approximately 2% of patients who receive heparin for more than 1 week. It is often associated with arterial microemboli and bleeding. As it is immunological, re-exposure to heparin will usually cause further problems. Severe thrombocytopenia may require withdrawal of heparin. A full blood count should be repeated regularly.

Other adverse effects

Osteoporosis may occur with prolonged high-dose therapy (e.g. 15 000 units/day for 6 months). Alopecia and hypersensitivity reactions may also occur. There is some evidence of adrenal suppression and so occasional plasma biochemistry should be assayed.

Warfarin (coumarin)

Warfarin antagonizes the effects of vitamin K and is the treatment of choice for long-term anticoagulation. Loading doses for 3–5 days are needed to achieve a steady state in most. It is conventional to start heparin for any indication that needs acute anticoagulation while allowing warfarin to take effect. Using warfarin initially may provoke a transient hypercoagulable state and heparin should balance this out.

Instituting treatment

Baseline clotting function (especially prothrombin time) should be measured. The usual initial dose for warfarin loading is 10 mg. A lower first dose, such as 5 mg, might be preferred in cases where the baseline prothrombin time is prolonged, the patient is on medications known to enhance the anticoagulant effect of warfarin, in elderly patients or those with low body weights and in patients with congestive cardiac failure or liver impairment.

A number of algorithms exist for warfarin loading but these were largely formulated in healthy subjects. However, a suitable one for general use is presented in Table 22.1.

Monitoring of treatment

Treatment is monitored by measuring the prothrombin time (PT) of the patient. Normally, this is expressed as a ratio of the PT of the patient to the PT of blood from an unanticoagulated patient as a control. This takes account of the sensitivity of the thromboplastin used to measure the PT. This ratio is known as the international normalized ratio (INR). If a loading dose of warfarin is to be used to achieve a rapid anticoagulation, then daily INR measurements are required for at least 4 days. Thereafter, once the INR is in the therapeutic range, measurements should be made weekly until the INR is stable and then

Table 22.1 Warfarin loading schedule [1].

Day	INR	Warfarin dose (mg)
First	< 1.4	10
Second	< 1.8	10
	1.8	1
	> 1.8	0.5
Third	< 2.0	10
	2.0–2.1	5
	2.2.-2.3	4.5
	2.4–2.5	4
	2.6–2.7	3.5
	2.8–2.9	3
	3.0–3.1	2.5
	3.2–3.3	2
	3.4	1.5
	3.5	1
	3.6–4.0	0.5
	> 4.0	0
Fourth (predicted maintenance dose)	< 1.4	> 8
	1.4	8
	1.5	7.5
	1.6–1.7	7
	1.8	6.5
	1.9	6
	2.0–2.1	5.5
	2.2–2.3	5
	2.4–2.6	4.5
	2.7–3.0	4
	3.1–3.5	3.5
	3.6–4.0	3
	4.1–4.5	Miss out next day's dose then give 2 mg
	> 4.5	Miss out 2 days' doses then give 1 mg

INR, international normalized ratio.

measurements can be less frequent, although should be at least every 3 months.

Target INR

The latest guidelines from the British Society of Haematology give target INRs for a range of clinical conditions [1]. A variation of 0.5 in the INR from the 'target' value is considered acceptable. These values are given in Table 22.2.

Adverse effects

Haemorrhage and/or excessive anticoagulation are the principal adverse effects of warfarin. Treatment of bleeding and/or excessive INR depends on

Table 22.2 Target international normalized ratios (INRs) for a range of clinical indications.

Indication	Target INR (allow ± 0.5 variation)
Pulmonary embolus, proximal or distal deep vein thrombosis, symptomatic inherited thrombophilia, atrial fibrillation (rheumatic, non-rheumatic, congenital heart disease, thyrotoxicosis), cardioversion, mural thrombus, cardiomyopathy	2.5
Recurrent deep vein thrombosis while on warfarin therapy, antiphospholipid syndrome, mechanical heart valve	3.5

Table 22.3 Management of bleeding and excessive anticoagulation.

Clinical problem	Action
Major bleeding	Stop warfarin Give prothrombin complex concentrate (50 units/kg) or FFP (15 mL/kg) Give 5 mg vitamin K (oral or i.v.)
INR > 8.0 No bleeding or minor bleeding	Stop warfarin Restart warfarin when INR < 5.0 If other risk factors for bleeding give 0.5–2.5 mg vitamin K (oral)
INR 6.0–8.0 No bleeding or minor bleeding	Stop warfarin Restart when INR 5.0
INR 4.0–6.0 target INR 3.5	Restart warfarin when INR < 5.0
INR 3.0–6.0 target INR 2.5	Restart warfarin when INR < 2.5

FFP, fresh frozen plasma; INR, international normalized ratio; i.v., intravenous.

the INR level and the extent of bleeding. Recommendations from the British Society of Haematology are shown in Table 22.3 [1].

Warfarin can rarely cause skin reactions, because of a mixture of skin necrosis and haemorrhage. Warfarin should not be used in pregnancy as it is teratogenic.

Interactions

Warfarin has a narrow therapeutic range and is affected by many common drugs. Any antiplatelet agent, NSAID or steroid may increase the incidence of gastrointestinal bleeding. Amiodarone increases the effects. Antibiotics that disrupt normal vitamin K production will allow the INR to climb rapidly. Any impairment or potentiation of liver function will affect INR; this includes alcohol binges and patients should be strongly advised not to have marked fluctuations in their alcohol intake. Appendix 1 of the *BNF* has a full list of interactions.

Anticoagulation of the surgical patient

Elective surgery

There are a number of factors to consider with regard to anticoagulation around the time of elective surgery.

Timing of cessation of warfarin preoperatively

If the patient is on warfarin because of a high risk of new clot formation or for the acute management of thromboembolic disease, then the INR should be allowed to correct by stopping warfarin 4–5 days before surgery. Typically, it takes 4 days for the INR to drop to 1.5 after cessation of warfarin [2].

Acceptable INR for surgery

This is very variable, although many surgeons require an INR of below 1.5 or 1.3 on the day of surgery. Local policy and preference should be established by consultation with the surgeon and anaesthetist.

Vitamin K is not generally used to correct the INR as this will disrupt the clotting cascade in an unpredictable fashion. It is important that the patient is aware that for a time he/she will not be fully anticoagulated and so will be at increased risk.

Alternative anticoagulation while warfarin is stopped

The use of heparin to cover the period of time when the patient is 'off warfarin' is dependent on a number of factors. One

of these factors is the indication for anticoagulation. The patient who is anticoagulated for atrial fibrillation as prophylaxis against stroke would be at very low risk for a short period of time without either warfarin or heparin cover. Many surgeons would find this acceptable, although some may suggest cover with aspirin in the perioperative period.

By contrast, a patient with a prosthetic valve should probably be switched onto intravenous UF heparin. However, it is worth noting that in a meta-analysis of studies covering a period of 53 647 patient-years in those with prosthetic heart valves, the risk of thromboembolic complication when not on warfarin was only 8 per 100 patient-years [3]. This translates into a risk of thrombosis of under 0.2% over a 7-day period without warfarin.

If heparin cover for the period of time without anticoagulation is preferred, then UF heparin should be started, usually when the INR falls below 2.0, and an APTT of 1.5–2.5 times control should be sought. The rate of infusion can be easily changed, stopped and restarted as required. It is for this reason that surgeons normally prefer it to LMW heparin. It is not normally given during the operation itself, typically being stopped 6 h preoperatively and recommenced 12 h postoperatively.

Emergency surgery

If the operation is urgent or an emergency then the risk–benefit ratio of anticoagulation may be substantially changed. Clotting may need to be reversed quickly using fresh frozen plasma (FFP) or platelets, depending on the advice of your local haematologist.

This provides cover for the procedure itself but is not likely to be sufficient postoperatively.

Unlike under elective conditions, vitamin K (1–10 mg) can be used with consideration of anticoagulation later. It will have an effect after 4–6 h. When using FFP, give 2–4 adult doses over 40 min to give transient control but this may not reverse high INRs for any long period. Check INRs twice a day on an unstable surgical patient on anticoagulation.

References

1 Guidelines on oral anticoagulation 3rd edn. *Br J Haematol* 1998; **101**: 374–87.

2 White RH, McKittrick T, Hutchinson R, Twitchell J. Temporary discontinuation of warfarin therapy: changes in the international normalized ratio. *Ann Intern Med* 1995; **122**: 40–2.

3 Cannegieter SC, Rosendaal FR, Briet E. Thromboembolic and bleeding complications in patients with mechanical heart valve prostheses. *Circulation* 1994; **89**: 635–41.

23: **Transfusion of blood products**

Transfusion of blood products is often necessary and can be immensely therapeutic if the correct product is used at the right time. It must always be remembered that any transfusion carries an element of risk and limiting this risk must be factored into every prescription.

Whole blood is donated by a generous population at a number of centres and mobile units throughout the country. Donors are excluded if they are from a high-risk group, if they have received a range of vaccinations, have a malignancy, use one or more of a specific list of drugs or have one or more of a variety of medical problems which are not considered further here. Each region has a transfusion depot to hold the reserves for its feeder hospitals. Each hospital also has a limited stock of blood products but can call upon the resources of the entire network in special circumstances. The consultant haematologist directs the use of blood products other than for the most simple red cell transfusions and should be consulted. All non-urgent blood donations will be cross-matched to the patient's antigen profile.

Whole blood is usefully separated out into red cells, plasma, platelets and the buffy coat of white cells. There can be further separations into specific clotting factors and albumin. In the past, blood transfusions have led to the transmission of human immunodeficiency virus (HIV) and hepatitis B and C. Blood is now routinely screened for viruses

including HIV. The recent bovine spongiform encephalopathy (BSE) epidemic and consequent new variant Creutzfeldt–Jakob disease (CJD) have cast doubt as to the safety of UK donated blood but there is no evidence of contamination as yet.

The most common call for blood products is the anaemic patient. While anaemia can have a number of definitions, probably the most useful is a reduction in oxygen-carrying capacity because of a low haemoglobin concentration in a patient with otherwise normal circulating volume. There is a normogram for haemoglobin concentration related to sex and age, but on average it is 11–13 g/dL for women and 12–15 g/dL for men.

A range of investigations should be carried out prior to any transfusion. The exact tests will depend on the individual case, but at least haemopoietic factors and a blood film should be performed.

Do not give blood to a person who has evidence of a chronic anaemia and is symptomless.

Common products, usage and special precautions

Whole blood

This is rarely used.

Packed red cells

These are stored chilled with citrate and glucose preservative. They have an acidic pH and so acid–base disturbances can be seen with massive transfusions. Each unit is approximately 330 mL. Packed cells can be given with a standard giving set in an emergency but it is better to use a proper blood-giving set with integral filter. Venflons greater than 20 G are advised.

Blood should be warmed if it is to be given as a rapid transfusion (at more than 50 L/min). Initially, small amounts should be given over 30 min in case of an adverse reaction. Give the entire unit over a maximum of 5 h. Minor pyrexia is common and is not an indication to stop. One unit of blood (usually 330 mL) increases the total haemoglobin concentration by 1 g/dL. It is rarely useful to give just a single unit and, if that is your intention, question the need.

Leucocyte-depleted blood

This is useful in immunocompromised patients. Use a filter as suggested by the blood bank. This can usually only be prescribed with the assent of the haematology department.

Fresh frozen plasma

This has the most humoral clotting factors and proteins. Its use is largely restricted to the treatment of any acute coagulopathy, e.g. bleeding secondary to warfarin therapy. The usual dose is 15 mL/kg. It may also be used as part of cycles of plasma exchange to replace clotting factors. Once thawed, it cannot be refrozen. It should be given quickly over 30 min. A normal giving set can be used with > 20-G cannula. (A bleeding patient should have larger access than this anyway.)

Cryoprecipitate

This is used if fibrinogen is low (< 2) following large volume transfusions.

The above products are usually given via a blood-giving set with an integral filter. The set does not need to be changed between doses of the same kind of fluid given sequentially, but a new set must be used every 12 h to guard against bacterial contamination.

Platelets

Pooled donor platelets are usually used, but occasionally single donor units are needed. Pooled donor platelets are less effective than single donor units. Generally, platelet transfusions should only be given if levels are below 50 and there is evidence of bleeding, or below 25 and a high risk of bleeding. In cases of immune-mediated consumption, such as thrombotic thrombocytopenic purpura (TTP), giving platelets may cause further problems by exposing antigenic targets and so the haematologist must be consulted before commencing therapy. A single adult dose is equivalent to 4–6 donations with a platelet content of 240×10^9 in a volume of approximately 300 mL. A fresh blood- or platelet-giving set primed with saline should be used. It does not need to be changed between sequential doses but should be discarded immediately after transfusion.

Albumin

This is extracted mostly from whole blood donation. It comes as 4–5 or 20% solutions. Its main use is in hypo-proteinaemic states with nephrotic syndrome or ascites and liver disease. Its role as volume replacement should be limited to states where low protein and oedema require salt and water restriction but there is a need for expansion of the circulating volume. There is some evidence that giving albumin in sepsis is associated with an increased overall mortality. It should be prescribed in the intravenous fluids section of the drug chart. The main use of 5% solution is in plasma expansion following burns and as part of plasma exchange.

Immunoglobulins

These are used to augment immunity to viruses and to achieve more rapid resolution of immune-mediated disease processes, such as Guillain–Barré syndrome and acute idiopathic thrombocytopenic purpura (AITP). The exact regimen forms part of specialist care and will not be considered further here. As with any such product, hypersensitivity is the main significant risk.

Prescribing issues

Blood products are usually prescribed in a separate section of the drug chart. Each unit should be written separately. If diuretics or other drugs are prescribed and intended to be given concurrently, this should be clearly stated in the same section but prescribed in the 'stat' section.

Problems with transfusions

In general, up to 20% of all transfusions are associated with adverse reactions.
Most are minor and the major ones occur usually as a consequence of clerical or administration error. Do not get frustrated with the nurse who wants to check the blood label thoroughly; it is vital and you should do it too.

Minor febrile reactions are common and are not indications to stop therapy. Occasionally, an acute haemolytic reaction is seen, usually because of an ABO incompatibility. Fever, back pain, hypotension and nausea are all early markers. If progressive, bleeding and organ damage ensue with fatal sequelae. Anaphylaxis-type reactions are also seen. If a compatibility reaction is suspected, stop the transfusion immediately and deal with any acute symptoms. Antihistamines and steroids may be needed. Contamination with viral or bacterial pathogens is rare but documented. The volume of fluid is often overlooked, and it is possible to induce heart failure by overload. In those at risk, a transfusion rate of around 1–2 mL/kg/h is advised. Diuretics can be used concomitantly. Massive transfusions may manifest electrolyte and clotting abnormalities. Potassium is slowly released from packed cells, while calcium is bound to stop clots forming. Rapid transfusions lead to a reduction in ionized calcium and hence myocardial damage. This can be prevented by giving 10 mL 10% calcium gluconate for every litre of citrated blood transfused. There are no platelets or clotting factors in packed red cells. Massive transfusions are associated with a dilutional coagulopathy. Clotting factors can be replaced with FFP or cryoprecipitate if necessary.

Checking a haemoglobin concentration immediately after transfusion may not be useful. Its main function is as a part of vigilance for continuing bleeding.

Examples of scenarios in which blood transfusion may be necessary

1 *Symptomatic anaemia with a cause under investigation.* Give blood slowly, having checked haematinics, etc. first.

2 *Asymptomatic anaemia with a cause under investigation.* If the picture is chronic, there is little merit in acute transfusion. However, make sure blood is available if needed.

3 *Acute bleed with normal haemoglobin.* Because of a delay in haemodilution, it is possible to have a normal value despite a significant bleed. Active bleeding with compromise should be treated aggressively. Any crystalloid or colloid will do (not 5% dextrose) for acute plasma expansion and O negative blood can be given if needed. Be prepared for large volume transfusion and cross-match immediately.

4 *Anaemia and heart failure.* The patient may benefit from increased oxygen-carrying capacity so give blood slowly and cover with diuretics if the fluid status is precarious.

The fastest way to obtain an estimate of haemoglobin is to perform a blood gas measurement on a venous or arterial sample.

For Jehovah's Witnesses the situation is a little problematic. This particular branch of Christianity has a core tenet that blood and blood products should not be taken into the body. This aspect of faith is protected by law and an enforced breach of this stated wish can be prosecutable. Most Witnesses carry a card to identify what, if any, blood product or fractions thereof they are willing to receive, e.g. immunoglobulins may be acceptable while red cells may not. A range of mechanisms and drugs are available to preserve blood loss intraoperatively and the senior members of the team should discuss this with the patient prior to any elective procedure. In the acute setting, synthetic plasma expanders should be used [1].

Emergency treatment

It is good practice to use fully cross-matched blood whenever possible. In an emergency, universal donor O Rhesus negative blood may be used. If more than 6 units have already been given, there is little merit in using fully matched blood. O negative blood is in very short supply and a cross-match sample should be sent immediately, which might allow the use of the more readily available O positive.

Reference

1 Muramoto O. Bioethical aspects of the recent changes in the policy of refusal of blood by Jehovah's Witnesses. *Br Med J* 2001; **322**: 37–9. [This paper in the education and debate section discusses the ethics and current changes in policy of refusal of blood products by Jehovah's Witnesses. It suggests that even if the religious status is clear, the attending doctor has a duty to clarify exactly what products can and cannot be used.]

24: The patient on steroids, the oral contraceptive pill or hormone replacement therapy

The adrenal cortex produces cortisol and aldosterone under a range of stimuli. The clinical use of replacement or supplemental corticosteroids is expanding. The dosage in individual situations will not be addressed further here; this chapter considers the principles of prescribing and conversion tables are presented.

Native cortisol (which is essentially hydrocortisone) has primarily glucocorticoid activity with some mineralocorticoid function. Aldosterone has almost entirely mineralocorticoid activity. Of the drugs listed in Table 24.1, hydrocortisone has the most mineralocorticoid activity with dexamethasone having the least. If true mineralocorticoid function is needed as part of a replacement regimen or to manage postural hypotension, fludrocortisone is used. This has negligible glucocorticoid activity. Prednisolone has primarily glucocorticoid function but also has moderate mineralocorticoid activity.

Use of steroids

The exact mechanism of action of corticosteroids in many disease states is not yet clear. Immunosuppressive and anti-inflammatory functions are probably most important. Corticosteroids are also used in conjunction with chemotherapy.

Mineralocorticoid adverse effects

Fludrocortisone and aldosterone affect renal tubular and collecting system water and sodium shifts. Water retention is the resultant effect but there may be significant sodium retention and hypertension, as in Conn's syndrome, with the simultaneous loss of potassium and alkalosis.

Glucocorticoid adverse effects

The side-effects of glucocorticoids are legion. Impaired glycaemic control, osteoporosis, proximal myopathy, psychoses, gastrointestinal bleeding and Cushing's syndrome are the most common and best known.

General adverse effects of steroids

Immunosuppression occurs and is often the mechanism by which the steroid is exerting its desired effect. This can lead to increased infections and a persistently elevated white count assay. Chickenpox is a particularly high risk and people on steroids may develop severe manifestations of the disease. Exposure to varicella zoster while on steroids is an indication for passive immunization with immunoglobulins.

Table 24.1 Relative glucocorticoid activity.

Drug	Dose (mg)	Routes of administration
Prednisolone	5	p.o., i.m.
Hydrocortisone	20	p.o., i.m., i.v., top
Dexamethasone	0.75	p.o., i.m., i.v.
Methylprednisolone	4	p.o., i.m., i.v.
Betamethasone	0.75	p.o., i.m., i.v.
Triamcinolone	4	i.m., intra-articular

i.m., intramuscular; i.v., intravenous; p.o., *per os* (oral); top, topical.

Maintenance treatment

Long-term prednisolone use should be at the lowest dose to maintain disease control, with this steady state being reviewed very regularly. Prophylaxis against osteoporosis and gastrointestinal bleeds should be employed.

Cessation of treatment

Prolonged use of glucocorticoids leads to the suppression of adrenal function because of what can be best described as atrophy. Dexamethasone diminishes corticotrophin secretion and this forms the basis of the dexamethasone suppression test for Cushing's syndrome.

The Committee on Safety of Medicines (CSM) advises a gradual withdrawal of steroids for those who have had prolonged (more than 3 weeks) use or repeated courses over a short interval. People at special risk are those who have taken the steroids in the evening. Taking nocturnal steroid has the biggest inhibitory effects on the pituitary–adrenal axis. To have the least effect, a large dose first thing in the morning is advised.

The formula for withdrawal is not strict. The endogenous levels of steroids are equivalent to 7–10 mg/day prednisolone. Assuming that the acute event has been adequately treated, the patient can be rapidly brought down to this level in stepwise fashion over a week and then by 1–2 mg every 3–5 days. Care must be taken over this period as relapses can occur and other events may supervene. Steroids should be increased in such cases and then withdrawn more slowly next time.

In cases of steroid-responsive COAD, the relapsing nature of the condition may require prolonged withdrawal over months. If steroid reversibility has not been tested, patients may have repeated courses of steroid unnecessarily with a resultant adrenal insufficiency state. Reducing the dose makes the patient feel unwell and may trigger a further acute attack, so making further prescription of steroids necessary and sadly unavoidable. This group will be very difficult to wean from exogenous steroid.

The surgical patient on steroids

The anaesthetist and surgeon must discuss the case fully. If there is inadequate steroid provision, marked hypotension can be seen at induction of anaesthesia. The postoperative period can be marred by cardiovascular instability, labile fluid status and poor healing.

If the patient has taken more than 10 mg/day of prednisolone equivalents for any duration within the preceding 3 months, supplemental steroids should be given preoperatively. For minor or day case procedures, this can be hydrocortisone prior to induction of anaesthesia with continuation of normal dosage afterwards. For longer procedures and those requiring a period of in-patient stay, normal steroids should continue, with intravenous hydrocortisone at the start of the operation and regularly thereafter for at least 72 h. Normal dosage (preoperative levels) should continue after this time with a gradual withdrawal as appropriate (Table 24.2). Methods of reducing the risk of adrenal suppression using prednisolone involve giving early morning doses and alternate day regimens.

Other issues

In the elderly or postmenopausal women, steroids at greater than 7.5 mg/day long term will accelerate osteoporosis. Bone loss is most evident within the first 6 months. In the majority, calcium and vitamin D supplements give adequate protection. If there is established osteoporosis or recent wrist or long limb fracture, bisphosphonates may have a role. Etidronate and alendronate are common choices for prevention of steroid-induced osteoporosis. Alendronate comes as a weekly dose of 70 mg. HRT is also used but should usually be avoided unless other symptoms of the menopause need treating also.

In pregnancy, long-term use of high doses can increase the risk of intrauterine growth retardation. There is little evidence for adrenal suppression in the fetus. Very small amounts will accumulate in breast milk at doses of less than 40 mg/day prednisolone. Dexamethasone crosses the placenta more readily and this should be taken into account when prescribing.

All patients taking steroids should be issued with a steroid information card. This is soft blue cardboard and has a steroid alert warning to inform patients, pharmacists and other health workers that the carrier has recently used or is still using steroids.

Hormone replacement therapy

HRT can be oestrogen alone (for women without an intact uterus) or combined oestrogen and progesterone (for those with a uterus). The progesterone helps prevent cystic hyperplasia of the endometrium that then progresses to malignancy. Progesterone is also needed if there are satellite endometrial foci after hysterectomy.

Benefits of and indications for HRT

HRT is useful in menopausal women

Table 24.2 Steroid replacement and surgery. When giving more than single doses of steroids in sick patients or those at high risk of gastrointestinal bleeds, H$_2$-blockers should be used or PPI if there has been a recent gastrointestinal bleed or active ulcer disease. Oral preparations of these should be used whenever possible.

Procedure	Morning of surgery	Preoperative	Postoperative	Follow-up
On steroids normally				
Major or long operation	Take normal morning dose or, if NBM, give hydrocortisone equivalent over 3 equal doses	Hydrocortisone 50 mg i.v. on induction	72 h of hydrocortisone 50 mg t.d.s. i.v. or 30 mg prednisolone orally	Continue maintenance steroids and withdraw normally if patient is well
Minor or day case	Take usual dose with usual medicines Taking double the usual dose the previous day is an acceptable alternative	Hydrocortisone 50 mg i.v. on induction	Back onto maintenance steroids	Continue maintenance steroids and withdraw normally if patient is well
Recently on steroids > 10 mg/day over last 3 months				
Minor or day case		Hydrocortisone 50 mg i.v. on induction	None	No maintenance
Major or long procedure		Hydrocortisone 50 mg i.v. on induction	72 h of hydrocortisone 50 mg t.d.s. i.v. or 30 mg prednisolone orally	No maintenance needed unless patient is ill and then slow withdrawal

NBM, nil by mouth.

with troublesome vasomotor symptoms (hot flushes) and vaginal atrophy. It is also useful in protecting against bone mass loss (osteoporosis), particularly in those who have undergone a hysterectomy with removal of the ovaries or non-surgical early menopause.

The usual duration of treatment with HRT is for 5 years. This confers the benefits of treatment while minimizing the risks (see below). In patients who have had a hysterectomy, treatment might be continued beyond 5 years, as they do not require progestogens and are not at risk of uterine neoplasia.

Risks of HRT

There is a very small increase in the incidence of breast cancer with long-term use of HRT (12 extra cases in 1000 with 15 years' use). There is a slight increase in the risk of DVT and these patients should ideally stop HRT 1 month before surgery. If not, then they should receive both mechanical and heparin DVT prophylaxis. A recent US study suggested an increased cardiovascular risk with long-term use although this remains controversial. This study group was using equine oestrogens and medroxyprogesterones.

HRT does not provide any contraception and indeed may allow fertility 1–2 years after the start of the menopause. If there is a possibility of pregnancy, barrier forms of contraception should be employed. If a patient has been on HRT for more than 10 years, its use should be reviewed.

Oral contraceptive pill

Oestrogen only, combined or progesterone only formulations of the OCP exist. In addition, depot progesterone forms are available for medium- and long-term use. (Section 7.3 of the *BNF* details the use of hormonal contraception.)

In many cases, the OCP can and should be continued while in hospital. However, if a patient has had a systemic upset, she may not be absorbing oral medication properly. Furthermore, she may have been prescribed enzyme-inducing drugs, reducing the efficacy of the OCPs and other methods of contraception should be used. It is very important to remind women of this while in hospital and it is probably prudent to document this advice.

The OCP (and indeed HRT) should be stopped immediately in thromboembolism or myocardial infarction, progressive or sudden hypertension, acute neuropsychiatric problems or CVA, liver dysfunction and pregnancy. It is prudent to stop oestrogen replacement or contraception 1 month prior to prolonged surgery, especially if there may be a period of immobility or reduced venous flow.

25: **Prescribing in organ failure**

Renal failure

Renal function is vital for the elimination of most endogenous waste products and exogenous drugs. Through its effects on fluid compartments, urea and proteins, renal function affects the volumes of distribution, levels of protein binding and plasma availability of drugs.

Renal failure is often described in terms of a biochemical assay of creatinine and creatinine clearance. This is used to calculate the glomerular filtration rate (GFR) but, without correction for age, sex and muscle bulk, values are misleading. For example, a frail elderly lady might have a normal creatinine in the high normal range. This value might lead to the assumption that she had a normal GFR but, in her, the anticipated creatinine should be much lower because of her lower body mass.

The Cockcroft–Gault formula can give an estimate of GFR. For women, the result should be multiplied by a factor of 0.85. This is only valid when renal function has been stable for a few days.

$$\underset{(mL/min)}{GFR} =$$
$$\frac{(140 - age) \times ideal\,body\,weight\,(kg)}{Serum\,creatinine\,(mg/dL) \times 72}$$

The GFR abnormality can be described as mild, moderate or severe and alterations in prescribing can be guided by this range. A GFR of less than 10 mL/min indicates severe impairment, 10–50 mL/min signifies moderate impairment and over 50 mL/min indicates mild or no impairment.

Renal clearance is not the only issue. The proximal tubule metabolizes many low molecular weight proteins such as insulin. Tubular dysfunction impairs this and explains the reduced insulin need for diabetics in renal failure. Oedema of the gut hampers absorption and elevated potassium augments the effects of digoxin. Uraemia affects platelet function and increases the bleeding risk in patients on warfarin. Uraemic toxins can also affect the hepatic cytochrome p450 and non-renal metabolism.

Loading doses

Loading doses are given to promote a rapid rise in plasma levels to obtain a steady state faster than by conventional regimens. This is especially important in drugs that have a long half-life. An important example of drug loading in renal failure is the use of digoxin for atrial fibrillation. Without a loading dose, steady state is achieved in a week. In renal failure, loading doses should be reduced by around 25%.

Maintenance doses

The total amount of drug given is influenced by the individual dose amount and the dosing interval. As a general rule, when high plasma levels are not needed, and there is a narrow therapeutic window, individual doses should be reduced; when high plasma levels are needed and the therapeutic range is wide, the dosing interval should be increased in renal failure. The latter approach results in greater oscillations of the plasma concentration. A combination of these approaches is usually adopted. Table 25.1 lists common drugs and an approach to dose adjustment based upon the estimated GFR is given.

Special cases

Diuretics

With the exception of spironolactone, diuretics act on the luminal side of the renal system and very high doses are needed to have the same clinical effect as seen in a patient without renal failure. When the GFR falls below 30 mL/min, thiazides have little effect on their own and loop diuretics should be used. If there is resistance to high-dose loop diuretics, this may be because of avoiding sodium retention downstream and the addition of a thiazide may be useful. Gut oedema will reduce absorption and the intravenous route is best used (see Diuretic section, Chapter 26).

NSAIDs

When renal perfusion is low, the glomerular filtration pressures have an increased dependence on renal prostaglandin vasodilators. These are inhibited by NSAIDs and lead to a precipitous—but reversible—fall in renal function. This class of drug will lead to tubular sodium retention and hence worsen any oedema and blunt the effects

of diuretics. They can be nephrotoxic in their own right and are best avoided in mild to moderate renal impairment. For patients on renal replacement therapy for irreversible disease, this precaution is less important.

Nephrotoxic drugs

Some drugs are toxic to the kidney at high doses. This is exaggerated in renal disease and such drugs are best avoided. If they are essential, very close monitoring is needed. Gentamicin is such an example.

Chronic renal failure

For patients who are on permanent renal replacement therapy, the need to protect against nephrotoxicity is less important; however, toxic levels are easily reached and great care is needed with prescribing. Despite best efforts, haemofiltration or dialysis cannot remove all endogenous agents so very careful monitoring is needed.

Liver failure

The liver is integral to the metabolism of most endogenous and exogenous substances. Metabolism can be described as phase 1 and phase 2. Phase 1 metabolism involves microsomal enzymes, with cytochrome p450 being one of the most commonly described. This provides the critical first hydroxylation step in the pathway for the metabolism of many drugs. Phase 2 involves conjugation to produce more hydrophilic complexes that can then be excreted in the urine or via the bile.

Table 25.1 Brief guide to drug dosage in renal failure [1].

Drug	Adjustment	Mild Dose (%)	Mild Interval (h)	Moderate Dose (%)	Moderate Interval (h)	Severe Dose (%)	Severe Interval (h)
Aciclovir*†	Dose/interval	100	12	100	12–24	50	24
Amoxicillin	Interval	100	8	100	8–12	100	12
Aspirin†	Interval	100	4–6	100	6–8	Avoid	
Atenolol	Dose	100	24	50	24	25	24
Carbamazepine*	Dose	100	12	100	12	75	12
Cefuroxime	Interval	100	8	100	12	50	12
Ciprofloxacin	Dose	100	12	50	12	33	12
Digoxin*	Dose/interval	75	24	50–75	24	25	24–48
Erythromycin	Dose	100	8	100	8	75	8
Gentamicin*†	Dose	70	24	50	24	25	24
Glibenclamide		100		Avoid		Avoid	
Lisinopril	Dose	100	24	50	24	25	24
Lithium CR*	Dose	100	24	50	24	25	24
Metformin‡		100		Avoid		Avoid	
Morphine	Dose	100	Vary	75	Vary	50	Vary
Piperacillin	Interval	100	6	100	8	75	8–12
Sotalol	Dose	100	12	50–30	12	15–30	12
Vancomycin	Interval	100	12–48	100	2–7 days	100	5–10 days
NSAIDs	Analgesic effects require no adjustment but can further compromise already impaired function. Best avoided						
Phenytoin*	Very close drug level monitoring needed with daily changes						
Frusemide	May need higher doses for diuretic effects						
Contrast	Can worsen renal failure						
Heparin/ warfarin	Dose adjustments depending on APPT/INR. Functional clotting may be off for other reasons so clinical vigilance is essential						

continued on p. 104

Table 25.1 (*continued*)

Drug	Adjustment	Mild		Moderate		Severe	
		Dose (%)	Interval (h)	Dose (%)	Interval (h)	Dose (%)	Interval (h)
Diltiazem Fluoxetine Tricyclics Valproate Amlodipine Amiodarone Haloperidol GTN Simvastatin	No adjustment needed for therapeutic levels but effects can be enhanced if using other similar acting drugs also						

APPT, activated partial thromboplastin time; GTN, glyceryl trinitrate; INR, international normalized ratio; NSAIDs, non-steroidal anti-inflammatory drugs.
* Monitor drug levels.
† Directly nephrotoxic.
‡ Risk of lactic acidosis.

Many drugs have biologically active metabolites, some of which are responsible for the adverse effect profile of the drug. In others, partial metabolism is essential for the therapeutic effect, e.g. paracetamol has its toxic metabolite following phase 1 metabolism.

In general terms, liver failure reduces drug metabolism and leads to drug accumulation. Portosystemic shunting further reduces first pass metabolism. If hepatic synthetic function is compromised, the resultant low protein state affects drug binding and a higher concentration of the free drug is observed. Hyperbilirubinaemia may also displace drugs from protein–binding sites and closer drug monitoring may be required in this circumstance.

First pass metabolism

This is metabolism of the drug following its absorption from the gut and passage

Table 25.2 Pro-drugs that are metabolized to active metabolites.

Pro-drug	Active metabolite
Heroin	Morphine
Codeine	Morphine
Azathioprine	Mercaptopurine
Enalapril	Enalaprilat
Diazepam	Nordiazepam

through the portal venous system, such that less active drug enters the systemic circulation. Drugs commonly affected by first pass metabolism include aspirin, chlorpromazine, GTN, levodopa, metoprolol, morphine, propranolol and verapamil.

Enzyme inducers and inhibitors

Many drugs are directly hepatotoxic.

Some induce liver enzymes, while others inhibit them. In general terms, the induction of liver enzymes increases drug metabolism and hence the clearance of drugs occurs at a faster rate. Rifampicin, alcohol, phenytoin and carbamazepine are examples of liver enzyme inducers (Table 25.2).

Reference

1 Schena FP. *Textbook of Nephrology*. McGraw-Hill, 2001.

26: **Drugs acting on the cardiovascular system**

The basics of prescribing cardiac drugs can be placed into categories: primary prevention, acute therapy and secondary prevention. The same drug classes are used in all categories.

Primary prevention

The Joint British Societies Coronary Risk Prediction Chart [1] is printed in the back of all new editions of the *BNF*. This tool is valuable in making predictions of the risks of developing cardiovascular system problems on the basis of risk factor profile. It is a primary prevention tool and anyone who has additive risk factors, such as a familial hypercholesterolaemia or diabetic end-organ disease, should be regarded in a high-risk group.

Acute management

The acute management of an unstable coronary syndrome, ST segment elevation myocardial infarction (STEMI) or non-STEMI is well described in almost every acute medical manual. This will not be repeated in detail here. Instead, the drugs commonly used are discussed with problems that may be encountered with each.

Secondary prevention

The National Service Framework for the management of cardiac disease has within it a range of recommendations that includes secondary prevention methods. From a purely prescribing aspect, this involves the use of antiplatelet drugs, statins, beta-blockers, spironolactone and ACE inhibitors when appropriate.

For the sake of clarity, this chapter does not try to reproduce the algorithms for therapy for every indication but instead concentrates on the drug classes involved and addresses prescribing issues. The information here is valid for any form of cardiovascular medicine including hypertension, stroke and heart failure.

Drug categories

Antiplatelet agents

Aspirin

There is a wealth of evidence for the use of aspirin. In primary prevention of stroke, 75 mg o.d. orally is beneficial. In acute myocardial ischaemia, 300 mg should be given initially followed by 75 mg o.d. Give 150 mg o.d. if the patient is already on aspirin. Unless there is active ulcer disease, this should be given orally to all patients. Enteric-coated, dispersible and rectal preparations exist but these have not been validated for this use, although they are likely to be of benefit.

Clopidogrel

This has less gastric irritation than aspirin but can still exacerbate gastrointestinal bleeding if there is an active ulcer or gastritis. The standard daily dose is 75 mg o.d. (300 mg loading dose). Clopidogrel is being increasingly employed in the acute setting in addition to aspirin if the patient was already on aspirin prior to admission. It can be used instead of aspirin where contraindications exist.

Glycoprotein IIb, IIIa inhibitors

These are licensed in the UK for the treatment of resistant unstable coronary syndrome while awaiting percutaneous transluminal coronary angioplasty (PTCA) or for post-PTCA management. They are used in combination with heparin and aspirin. The NICE suggests that they should be used widely but, at present, their use is limited to specialist centres only. There is a significant risk of bleeding.

Thrombolytics

Thrombolytics should be given as soon as possible after the start of an STEMI and certainly within 12 h. There are audit standard times for thrombolysis in hospitals and most have measures in place to ensure treatment within 20 min of arriving at hospital. Streptokinase, alteplase (tpA), reteplase and tenecteplase are available. All are given intravenously (Table 26.1).

Active severe bleeding or recent acute haemorrhagic stroke are absolute contra-indications. Severe hypertension should be treated first as the risk of a stroke is very high. In pregnancy, there is a risk of placental separation and fetal haemorrhage (see Chapter 9).

Table 26.1 List of common thrombolytics used in myocardial infarction.

Initial dose	Interval dose	Heparin	Approx. cost (£)	Sequelae
Streptokinase 1.5 units over 60 min	None	No	90	Antibodies seen after 4 days
Alteplase (rt-PA) 10 mg bolus	50 mg over 60 min 40 mg over 120 min	Yes	600	
Reteplase 10 units over 2 min	10 units over 2 min, 30 min later	Yes	720	
Tenecteplase 500 micrograms/kg (max 50 mg) over 10 s	None	Yes	770	

Low molecular weight heparins

Dalteparin and enoxaparin are used in acute coronary syndromes. These are given subcutaneously twice a day. Dalteparin 120 units/kg (maximum 100 000 units) or enoxaparin 100 units/kg are commonly used agents in this category. There is yet to be a consensus on the use of LMW heparin after thrombolysis.

Unfractionated heparin

The use of unfractionated heparin in unstable angina has now been superseded but it retains a place where there may be a bleeding risk and close monitoring of levels is available. It is also sometimes used for post-thrombolysis therapy. While high-dose twice daily subcutaneous regimens exist (12 500 units b.d. s.c. for mural thrombus), heparin is still commonly given as an intravenous infusion. The APTT should be 2–3 times the control (see Heparin in Chapter 22).

Prefilled heparin syringes or bottles with a set concentration exist. Watch for hyperkalaemia and thrombocytopenia.

Beta-blockers

The class is fairly heterogeneous in the selectivity and specificity of action at the $beta_1$ cardiac adrenoceptors. Some have a peripheral vasodilating element to their profile due to mixed alpha and beta effects. Others have partial agonist function and cause less bradycardia and less vasoconstriction (normally unopposed alpha activity).

When choosing and prescribing beta-blockers, therapy should be thought of as acute or long-term. For acute intravenous use as in peri-MI, rhythm disturbances and hypertension, short-acting agents are advised. For those with reactive airways, highly cardioselective agents may be employed if absolutely essential but regular checks of lung function are needed. In peripheral vascular disease, vasodilating or cardioselective agents are more suitable. Beta-blockers can cause hallucinations and nightmares and in susceptible patients water-soluble agents should be chosen, as these do not cross into the brain as easily. In renal failure, water-soluble drugs can accumulate and a dose reduction is needed.

Most agents can be taken orally once a day but twice or three times daily preparations can be used to exploit the side-effects and treat the somatic features of anxiety or depression. This is also the case for acute migraine and hyperthyroidism. Here, propranolol, which is lipid soluble, has an enduring role. If treating hypertension, monotherapy is usually not enough. Combination with a thiazide diuretic in the first instance is advised. Other drugs may also be needed. If palpitations and high blood pressure are caused by a phaeochromocytoma, alpha-blockade is needed concurrently.

Bisoprolol and carvedilol are licensed for cardiac failure, but long-acting metoprolol is also sometimes prescribed. This should be initiated in hospital under supervision. The lowest oral dose of the chosen drug is given with blood pressure monitoring every 10–20 min. A clinical review is needed within 2 weeks and an increase in dosage should be given if there are no problems.

Table 26.2 lists common beta-blockers with a basic scoring system. Despite the differences, all beta-blockers

Table 26.2 Beta-blockers available.

Drug	Beta$_1$ selectivity	Acute use in MI	ISA	Vasodilates	Use in heart failure	Water soluble	Main use
Atenolol	++	++	−	−	−	+++	IHD, hypertension
Bisoprolol	++	+	−	−	++	+	IHD, heart failure
Carvedilol	+	−	+	+	++	+	Heart failure
Metoprolol	−	++	−	−	+		IHD, hypertension
Sotalol	+	−				+++	Rhythm disturbances
Propranolol	−	+	−	−	−	−	Rhythm disturbances, anxiety state
Esmolol	+	−	−	−	−	−	Acute rhythm disturbances
Labetalol	−	−	−	++	−	−	Hypertension
Nebivolol	−	−	+	++		+++	IHD, hypertension
Celiprolol	+	−	−	+	−	+	Hypertension

IHD, ischaemic heart disease; ISA, intrinsic sympathomimetic activity; MI, myocardial infarction.
−, Effect not seen or possibly harmful; +, effect seen and beneficial.

will reduce cardiac output. They should be stopped if hypotension is seen, especially if there is an intercurrent illness leading to shock. The most common side-effect is fatigue. Reduced libido and impotence can also be seen. In smokers, check PEFR at the start of therapy and for a few days thereafter. In diabetics, there is some reduction in the sensations of hypoglycaemia, but the benefits of good beta-blockade are often greater. The traditionally recommended use of bisoprolol over other agents in hyperlipidaemic patients is based on limited data only.

There is evidence that beta-blockade given acutely reduces mortality in MI. This is especially so in large anterior infarcts when the risk of ventricular rupture is greater. Give atenolol 5 mg i.v. or metoprolol 10–25 mg over 5 min and repeat every 15–20 min. Oral agents can be substituted at the next convenient dose. The arbitrary marker for adequate beta-blockade is a stable resting heart rate of 60 b.p.m. or less.

Lipid regulating agents

The guidelines are always shifting here

but the current suggestions are that all IHD patients should be on a statin as part of secondary prevention for IHD, whatever the cholesterol value and relative ratio of high-density lipoprotein (HDL) to low-density lipoprotein (LDL). There is considerable evidence that reducing the total cholesterol below 5 mmol/L (or by 25%) or LDL by about 30% is useful in primary prevention in at-risk but asymptomatic groups. This value is under constant challenge and may have already changed by publication.

Anion exchange resins

These bind bile acids and lead to a reduction in LDL cholesterol by up-regulating LDL receptors in the liver. A paradoxical rise in triglycerides is sometimes seen. Constipation is the most common side-effect.

Fibrates

These act across the spectrum but have a greater effect on lowering triglyceride levels. Their use is largely restricted to mixed hyperlipidaemias.

Statins

These inhibit HMG-CoA reductase and so reduce liver cholesterol synthesis. They have a significant effect on lowering LDL cholesterol, raising HDL cholesterol and some slight reduction on triglyceride levels. In the acute setting, anti-inflammatory and plaque stabilizing effects may affect the morbidity and mortality to a greater extent than as a consequence of the lower cholesterol level. There is probably no need to give these at night time as often stated.

Liver disease or excess alcohol are contra-indications. Liver function should be checked prior to starting therapy and twice a year thereafter. Myositis is well reported, although rare, and a patient with any unusual muscle symptoms should have liver function and creatine kinase assays and their statin should be stopped. A transient asymptomatic threefold rise in transaminase concentration is acceptable, but not if it persists.

There is much publicity surrounding the various statins available but most of the published evidence on improvements in mortality and morbidity relates to the use of simvastatin. Other studies have looked at the measurement of absolute values of cholesterol and these data are probably safe to extrapolate.

ACE inhibitors

ACE inhibitors have proven especially useful in all forms of IHD and hypertension therapy. They should be given to the majority for secondary prevention and there is some evidence that they have a role in primary prevention of 'high-risk groups', especially if the subject is diabetic.

Their role is in reducing pre- and after-load but the presence of angiotensin II receptor populations in endothelium, adipose tissue and a number of organ systems suggests functions that have yet to be adequately defined.

ACE inhibitors have a potassium-sparing function and should be used with caution in combination with potassium supplements and potassium-sparing diuretics. In renal failure, the effect on pre- and post-capillary vaso-motor tone alters the GFR and can make renal impairment worse. They are contra-indicated in renal artery stenosis and are generally best avoided in any form of renovascular disease.

The widely held belief that everyone should have a captopril trial is false. This was initially suggested to observe the phenomenon of 'first-dose hyperten-sion', which may be seen if the patient is also taking high-dose loop diuretics or is underfilled. This can be seen with all members of the class and captopril has a shorter half-life making it more suitable for this 'test'. As long as adequate super-vision is available and simple checks on volume state and renal function are made, there is no reason to use a different agent from that planned for long-term therapy.

Most ACE inhibitor treatment is given once a day but high doses for the treatment of heart failure or post-MI are sometimes divided. Captopril should be given in 2–3 divided doses. Assuming normal renal function and adequate circulating volume, the lowest dose on the formulary on the 'one-off' section of the drug chart should be prescribed at a specific time. Blood pressure should be checked on giving the drug, at 30 min and then hourly for 4 h after that. A drop in blood pressure is expected, and first-dose hypotension is not an indication to stop ACE inhibitors, but a precipitous symptomatic fall indicates marked sensi-tivity. Angiotensin II receptor blockers may be more useful in some such cases. If the blood pressure change is safe, doses are increased as per *BNF* guidelines to the maximum tolerated.

The main reason for lack of compli-ance is a persistent dry cough. This symptom does not resolve with time in most and a change in drug class to an an-giotensin II inhibitor may be indicated. Angio-oedema is a major adverse effect and ACE-I should be avoided if there has been a history of this.

Angiotensin II receptor antagonists

These are given twice a day and are used as an alternative to ACE-I where side-effects are troublesome. They are occa-sionally used in conjunction with ACE-I for the treatment of heart failure.

Calcium-channel blockers (referred to incorrectly as calcium antagonists)

These have an additive role in the treat-ment of angina by reducing cardiac work. The evidence that there is a long-term improvement in mortality is limited. They are not useful in acute angina unless as a consequence of coro-nary vasospasm. However, they are an important element in the management of hypertension and rhythm disturbances.

As with beta-blockers, the group is fairly heterogeneous with the three prin-cipal groups having different effects on heart rate, contractility and peripheral resistance. These are dihydropyridines (amlodipine, nifedipine, nimodipine), phenylalkamines (verapamil) and benzothiapines (diltiazem). They can all cause bradycardia and should be avoided in any heart block.

Dihydropyridines

Nifedipine is a short-acting agent that has a greater effect on peripheral and cardiac vascular tone. It has minor negative inotropic function and negligible effects on heart rate. Like other drugs in its group it is a poor antiarrhythmic. Because of unpredictable effects on blood pressure, it is not advised for angina or hypertension, although long-acting preparations are still used for this purpose. Amlodipine and felodipine are similar but have even less effect on contractility and so can be used in heart failure. These are naturally long-acting agents and are given once a day. Nimodipine is restricted to use in cerebrovascular spasm following a subarachnoid bleed, where it has a preferential action.

Phenylalkamines

Verapamil is the only drug in clinical use in its class. It is a potent negative chronotrope and inotrope. It has a role in rapidly achieving rate control in supraventricular tachycardias but can also precipitate heart failure. It should be used with extreme caution with beta-blockers (preferably, not at all) because of the additive effects on rate and contractility.* Oral, intravenous and long-acting preparations exist. It is still used as an antihypertensive by some but this is becoming less common.

Verapamil has been largely superseded but is used for rhythm and rate disturbances. The intravenous dose is 5–10 mg given slowly (2 min) and repeated after 10–20 min. Very close mon-

itoring is needed. The oral dose is 40–120 mg t.d.s. as an antiarrhythmic and 80–120 mg t.d.s. as an antianginal and antihypertensive. Long-acting preparations also exist.

Benzothiapines

These block the L-type calcium channel preventing calcium influx during myocardial and smooth muscle contraction. There is a prolonged refractory period in the AV node. The result is a relaxation of vascular tone and drop in blood pressure and a slower and weaker cardiac cycle. They are metabolized in the liver at first pass and used in a three times daily regimen. Long-acting preparations exist that give a much smoother effect on measurable parameters of rate and blood pressure and these should be used in preference to the pure drug when possible.

Diltiazem is usually used in angina or hypertension when rate control is needed and there is a contra-indication to beta-blockade. The starting dose is 60 mg t.d.s. but can be increased threefold if necessary. Long-acting preparations are preferred once it is clear that the patient tolerates the drug well.

From Table 26.3, it is apparent that amlodipine has a place when hypertension and heart failure exist. It is useful for the treatment of isolated systolic hypertension commonly seen in the elderly. The starting dose is 5 mg with a maximum of 10 mg/day.

Generally, if a patient presents in heart failure or with conduction abnormalities, stop calcium-channel blockers immediately and arrange an assessment of cardiac function after a wash-out period.

---

* The intravenous preparation of verapamil and beta-blockers should not be combined as asystole can occur.

Table 26.3 The characteristics of calcium-channel blockers.

Drug	Effects on rate	Effects on contractility	Vasomotor tone	Angina	BP	Antiarrhythmic	Safe in heart failure
Verapamil	++++	++++	+	++	+	+++	−
Diltiazem	++	++	++	++	++	++	−/+
Amlodipine	−	−	++	+	+++	+	+

Beta-blockers and potent calcium-channel blockers used together can induce heart failure, extreme bradycardia and even asystole

Nitrates and potassium-channel openers

Nitrates (oral, sublingual, buccal, transcutaneous or intravenous) work by providing a source of nitric oxide which is a potent vasodilator. There is no evidence that nitrates improve mortality but they have a clear and reproducible effect on symptoms. Their main effects are on coronary vessels and venous capacitance. There is some effect on intracerebral arteries, and also peripheral arterial resistance. This results in a reduction in pre-load, which reduces intramural tension, and an improvement in myocardial oxygenation, especially at the subendocardial level. There is a drop in blood pressure because of reduced output and reduced resistance. The main side-effect is severe headache. Tachyphylaxis is commonly seen with the use of nitrates and a gradual increase in dosage requirements is often required after prolonged use. It is for this reason that a nitrate-free period is advised if at all possible and the lowest dose tolerated should be used at all times.

The use of nitrates can be separated into acute symptom control, as part of therapy for on-going ischaemia, and rapid reduction of pre-load and afterload in heart failure and the management of hypertension.

Preparations of nitrates

Nitrates are available in many forms including glyceryl trinitrate (GTN), isosorbide dinitrate (ISDN) and isosorbide mononitrate (ISMN). GTN provides rapid symptom relief and comes in several preparations.

GTN sublingual tablets are available as 300- and 500-microgram tablets. They work almost immediately and have an effect for around 20 min. They have a shelf life of only 8 weeks and should be discarded after that. Check if the date is valid if patients report increasing GTN use.

Aerosol sprays contain 400 microgram per dose and bottle sizes vary. Use 1–2 sprays for acute symptom relief, working in seconds. This can be repeated a number of times but convention is that more than three times in an hour should prompt a call for help as it suggests continuing ischaemia. The preparations are more stable and have a much longer shelf life of 4–6 months.

Buccal preparations come as 1-, 2-, 3- and 5-mg sustained-release tablets. The tablet should be placed high up between upper lip and gums. There will be some swallowing of the agent but this does not cause any problems. In acute severe angina or heart failure, 5 mg can be used as an alternative to the intravenous route. The intravenous route is preferred in severe angina or acute heart failure and hypertension.

1 Make 50 mg GTN up to 50 mL with normal saline or 5% dextrose. Predilut-ed bottles exist at this concentration.*

2 The usual dosage range is from 0 to 10 mg/h with a titration to response.

3 For angina, start at 2 mg/h and in-crease in a stepwise manner until symptom control is achieved. Nitrates are given at the same time as other acute therapies including opiates.

4 Once there has been a period of stability for an hour, reduce the infusion rate as tolerated. Give the lowest dose to provide symptom control. This reduces the incidence of tolerance developing.

For heart failure, start the infusion at 2 mg/h and increase until the blood pressure falls. Here the emphasis is to reduce pre- and after-load. For hyper-tension, establish a level to be achieved and titrate the dose in 1-mg steps. There will be a differential drop in systolic and diastolic levels. In most cases of hyper-tension needing acute intervention, the diastolic should be largely maintained in order to perfuse the coronary vessels (see Chapter 27).

ISDN and ISMN are more stable and are better suited for oral administration, although they are also available in other forms. Transdermal nitrate patches provide a 24-h sustained release and are useful if long-acting oral preparations cannot be used. As a constant back-ground of nitrate is given, tachyphylaxis will rapidly develop.

For the long-acting oral preparations, the mechanism of sustained release should guide use. Some are twice daily preparations and should be given to allow a nitrate-free period; others are once a day with this factor built in. The time when a significant number of pre-cariously balanced patients suffer pain is first thing in the morning and so regi-mens should take this into account. Short-acting sprays or tablets can be used at the same time as patches or sus-tained release tablets but this suggests a worsening of symptoms and a medical review is needed.

When first using nitrates, check if there is a fixed cardiac performance problem such as aortic stenosis as a severe fall in cardiac output may ensue. Warn the patient of headaches and flush-ing: 'This is evidence the drug is working'. The first dose can cause hy-potension and so it is worthwhile to demonstrate the use of the spray or tablet in a controlled environment.

For frequent exertional angina, pro-phylactic use 5–10 min before an activity can help. Sustained release nitrates can also be used in the management of chronic heart failure as adjuvant therapy to reduce pre-load but should not be used to treat hypertension.

---

* Use polyethylene syringes if possible, as the common PVC type causes the effects to decay. Many units have a 24-h discard policy instead, which makes less financial sense.

Nicorandil

Nicorandil is the first of the commercially available potassium-channel openers licensed for use in IHD. It dilates epicardial and subendocardial coronary vessels and has a nitrate-like effect with a reduction in pre-load. Recent evidence has supported its use in the management of unstable angina. Its other effect is in mimicking cardiac preconditioning, a phenomenon in which the area of ischaemia appears to reduce with repeated submaximal ischaemic stimuli. The dose is 5–30 mg b.d. orally. It is not widely accepted for monotherapy as yet, although evidence is accumulating for this, and it is usually regarded as second- or third-line add-on therapy.

Thiazide and loop diuretics

These are used in a range of situations including hypertension and heart failure. They are discussed below and in Chapter 27. Thiazide diuretics (bendrofluazide (bendroflumethiazide), hydrochlorathiazide, metolazone) act on the distal convoluted tubule preventing sodium uptake and hence inducing a diuresis. They act within 2 h of administration and last for 24 h. They are the first-line drug of choice in hypertension and should be used as part of the treatment regimen for heart failure. The diuretic effect of bendrofluazide is modest. Its efficacy in hypertension at 2.5 mg is probably because of effects on vascular smooth muscle. There is little merit in using other forms for hypertension.

Metolazone is particularly useful in combination with a loop diuretic in causing a large volume diuresis. It should be given 20 min prior to the loop diuretic (usually frusemide). It is best used as a twice daily regimen, initially at 5–10 mg/day.

Loop diuretics (frusemide, bumetanide) act on the ascending limb of the loop of Henle to prevent sodium and hence water uptake. They are potent diuretics, especially at first exposure. Bumetanide is 40 times more potent than frusemide at the same dose. Both drugs work within 60 min of oral intake and have an effect sustained for up to 6 h (so a proprietary name for frusemide is *Lasix*). Intravenous preparations are available and they can also be given intramuscularly.

Very high doses may be needed in renal failure or resistant heart failure. Hypokalaemia is a feature of both classes, especially if combined. The resultant diuresis may lead to a lower circulating volume state and hence postural hypotension. Daily weights are a better marker of total fluid load than fluid charts, and weight charts should be used if treating congestive cardiac failure. In severe congestive cardiac failure, gut oedema impairs absorption and so the intravenous route is chosen. Bumetanide may be slightly better absorbed from the gut and therefore has a preferential use in such cases.

Giving diuretics late in the day causes unnecessary worry and nocturnal urinary frequency. A twice daily regimen of frusemide should be given in the early morning and early afternoon (6 a.m. or 8 a.m., and 2 p.m.). Thiazides should be given first thing in the morning.

Potassium-sparing diuretics

Amiloride and triamterene are weak

diuretics and are best used in combination with other drugs. They help in retaining potassium but can lead to hyperkalaemia and so regular monitoring is still needed. Combination drugs incorporating these with other diuretics are on the market and widely used. For stable patients in the community, these may be appropriate.

Spironolactone antagonizes the effects of aldosterone. It is a moderate diuretic and also retains potassium. It too is best used in combination with another agent. In heart failure, a combination of low-dose spironolactone 25 mg, an ACE inhibitor and a loop diuretic has been shown to improve mortality and morbidity. Its other major use is in the treatment of oedema and ascites of cirrhosis.

Reference

1 *Heart* 1998; **80**: S1–29.

27: **Hypertension**

Definition of hypertension

Hypertension has been defined in a number of different ways. The Framington study took a blood pressure of 160/95 mmHg to be abnormal and a blood pressure of between 140/90 and 160/95 mmHg as borderline [1]. Meanwhile, the WHO-ISH guidelines suggest that 140/90 mmHg and above represents hypertension [2]. On an individual basis, it can be a level above which there is greater good than harm from reduction. The Joint Consultative Committee on Hypertension has given us a practical value of 140/80 mmHg for the majority of the adult population as the cut-off for hypertension.

Patients in hospital manifest high blood pressure for a number of reasons:
1 The blood pressure may not have been taken correctly (is the cuff size correct for the patient?).
2 The patient is in a stressful environment and ill.
3 The patient has not taken his/her medications correctly.
4 The patient is normally hypertensive but no-one has noticed this before.

The management of hypertension is difficult and is very much based on local practice in spite of the range of guidelines available. It is vital to remember that a blood pressure reading is merely a number and has limited value unless taken in the context of the patient and previous readings. A known hyperten-sive patient who has not had medications for a few days and has a systolic value of 120 mmHg has either been suddenly cured or is relatively hypotensive from another cause. Organ autoregulation may have adjusted to respond to higher pressures and so any period of relative hypotension may be associated with significant underperfusion of organs, especially the kidneys.

Stepwise approach to the treatment of hypertension

The initial treatment of hypertension should include a reduction in risk factors, including weight reduction, stopping smoking, increasing physical exercise and a reduction in salt intake. In more stable cases of essential hyperten-sion, there should be a stepwise increase in pharmacological therapy. There are many different potential treatments for hypertension. Three long-term studies comparing the major classes of antihy-pertensive drugs have been published and have shown no significant difference in efficacy, side-effects or improvement in quality of life [3–5].

Commonly-used classes are as follows with examples. See section on cardio-vascular drugs for further prescribing information.
1 *Low-dose thiazides:* (e.g. bendroflu-azide 2.5 mg o.d. orally) should be first line in straightforward cases of essential hypertension.

2 *ACE-I* (ramipril 10 mg o.d. orally) or angiotensin II inhibitors (e.g. losartan 50 mg b.d. orally).

3 *Beta-blockers:* bisoprolol 10 mg o.d. orally.

4 *Calcium antagonists:* amlodipine 10 mg o.d. orally, especially useful in isolated systolic hypertension in the elderly.

5 *Alpha-blockers:* doxazosin 8 mg orally.

6 *Centrally acting agents:* moxonidine 600 micrograms orally in divided doses.

More than one agent is usually needed and this allows for lower doses of each class.

In addition to general health measures and the treatment of hypertension, the use of aspirin and statins to reduce cardiovascular risk factors further should be considered. The Joint British Societies Coronary Risk Prediction Chart is at the back of the *BNF*. This stratifies the likely risks of heart disease and helps to guide therapy.

Perioperative blood pressure control

If a patient is significantly hypertensive prior to anaesthesia, a sudden and profound hypotension may occur at the time of induction. Relative hypertension may be seen on recovery from anaesthesia. For this reason, the blood pressure and volume status of all patients should be optimized prior to any operation. For elective procedures, patients should take all cardiac medications as normal prior to the operation. A recent measurement of urea and electrolytes should also be available.

Hypertension in the immediate preoperative period may result from anxiety. A short-acting low-dose anxiolytic, such as temazepam 10–20 mg orally, may be useful. This should probably be avoided in the day case unit as patients may be quite sleepy after what may have been a short procedure.

In the postoperative period, hypertension is often a reflection of pain and/or a lack of normal medications. These should be addressed. While for the vast majority temporary mild hypertensive episodes are unlikely to do harm, in certain states a very tight control of blood pressure is needed, e.g. vascular surgery and neurosurgery. Many centres will have local protocols for managing these patients.

Acute control of blood pressure

This is sometimes essential and can be performed using nitrates, alpha- and beta-adrenoceptor antagonists intravenously. Short-acting dihydropyridines (nifedipine crush) are no longer advised.

Nitrates

The formulation for GTN is as described in Chapter 26.

Adrenoceptor antagonists

Intravenous beta-adrenoceptor antagonists can be used with care. These act mainly by reducing cardiac output and through a renal adaptive mechanism and not vasodilatation. The use of these drugs requires full cardiac monitoring facilities in the presence of appropriately trained staff. There are a number of alternatives for intravenous beta-adrenoceptor antagonists. It is most appropriate to define not only the drug dose, concentration and the duration of therapy, but also a sliding scale of treatment relative to blood pressure. Sensitivity to these drugs varies substantially between individuals and so a small test dose is often advisable. If the patient is a smoker or there is any evidence of airways disease, it may be useful to measure PEFR prior to starting treatment. This may need to be repeated while the treatment becomes established.

Clonidine has alpha-adrenoceptor blocking activity. It is a useful short-term intravenous antihypertensive (150–300 micrograms over 24 h) and also has some anxiolytic activity, although the mechanism of this is uncertain and may be related to transiently altered central noradrenaline activity. It is now rarely used for long-term therapy and care must be taken as rebound hypertension can be very marked on cessation of treatment. If it is used, close monitoring of blood pressure is required.

Issues in prescribing antihypertensive medications

Thiazide diuretics

Bendrofluazide is a thiazide diuretic that has its antihypertensive effects at 2.5 mg because of its effects on vascular tone. This has a flat dose–response curve, so higher doses are not usually beneficial. If a true diuresis is desired, a loop diuretic is more appropriate. Thiazides will deplete sodium and potassium and so regular checks are advised.

Loop diuretics

Frusemide is a very powerful loop diuretic. It also has significant effects on smooth muscle relaxation. In isolation, diuretics are not good antihypertensives. Prescribing diuretics after 6 p.m. causes unnecessary distress and night disturbance.

ACE inhibitors

ACE inhibitors result in an improvement in survival greater than the benefit that might be expected from the effects of the ACE inhibitor on blood pressure alone. There are a range of receptor subtypes distributed in muscle, fat, endothelium, heart and brain and it is thought that these may be responsible for the observed benefits of these drugs. They have a potassium-sparing effect and potassium supplements and potassium-sparing diuretics should be stopped prior to starting ACE inhibitor treatment.

There may be marked first-dose hypotension with ACE inhibitors. Initiation of therapy is described in Chapter 26.

Diabetic patients in particular may benefit from using ACE-I as first-line therapy.

Beta-blockers

Once daily beta-blockers can be given at night time so that the effects are seen by the morning ward round. Traditionally, a resting heart rate of above 60 b.p.m. suggests inadequate beta-blockade.

Calcium-channel blockers

Calcium-channel blockers have differing effects on blood pressure and cardiac output. Caution should be employed if using in combination with other negative inotropes and negative chronotropic drugs. Do not use short-acting agents such as nifedipine for the control of systemic blood pressure.

References

1 Gordon T, Castelli WP, Hjortland MC, Kannel WB, Dawber TR. Predicting coronary heart disease in middle-aged and older persons. The Framington Study. *J Am Med Assoc* 1977; **238**: 497–9.

2 Chalmers J, MacMahon S, Mancia G *et al*. The 1999 WHO-ISH Guidelines for the Management of Hypertension. *Clin Exp Hypertens* 1999; **21**: 1009–60.

3 Neaton JD, Grimm RH, Prineas RJ *et al*. Treatment of mild hypertension study: final results. Treatment of Mild Hypertension Study Research Group. *J Am Med Assoc* 1993; **270**: 713–24.

4 Materson BJ, Reda DJ, Cushman WC *et al*. Single-drug therapy for hypertension in men: a comparison of six antihypertensive agents with placebo. The Department of Veterans Affairs Cooperative Study Group on Antihypertensive Agents. *N Engl J Med* 1993; **328**: 914–21.

5 Philipp T, Anlauf M, Distler A, Holzgreve H, Michaelis J, Wellek S. Randomised, double blind, multicentre comparison of hydrochlorothiazide, atenolol, nitrendipine, and enalapril in antihypertensive treatment: results of the HANE study. HANE Trial Research Group. *Br Med J* 1997; **315**: 154–9.

28: **Cardiac arrhythmias**

The precise nature of any cardiac arrhythmia must be established before treatment can be undertaken. Clinical examination will help and a 12-lead electrocardiogram (ECG) is essential. An important distinction is between supraventricular and ventricular arrhythmias.

Classification of drugs

Antiarrhythmics work by slowing conduction or prolonging a refractory phase, stabilizing excitable membranes, reducing effects of circulating catecholamines or enhancing vagal tone. Combining agents of different classes can precipitate conduction abnormalities and even syncope. Most antiarrhythmics can cause most types of rhythm disturbance at high plasma levels.

The Vaughan Williams classification of antiarrhythmics is still used widely. However, it is far from exhaustive and many newer agents do not fall into this system easily (Table 28.1).

Important drugs used in arrhythmias

Amiodarone*

This is a class III drug that has the

calcium antagonist effects of rate control and myocardial depression, and antiarrhythmic properties greater than beta-blockade. It has a role in the management of most arrhythmias. Its main problems are unpredictable effects on thyroid function (both hyper- and hypothyroidism) because of the iodine it contains, a rise in liver transaminases and, most importantly, pulmonary fibrosis. More noticeable effects are skin discoloration, corneal microdeposits and photosensitivity. These should all be fully discussed prior to therapy and baseline liver function and thyroid function should be measured. Worsening respiratory function is a marker of lung disease that may not be entirely reversed on stopping the drug.

The pharmacological properties of amiodarone are not fully understood. There is no widespread consensus for a good loading regimen. This is largely because it has a very long half-life. Once a good loading level is achieved, minor day-to-day alterations make little difference. It can be given as intravenous or oral preparations and can be crushed to be used via a nasogastric tube.

It now features in the advanced life support (ALS) algorithm for resuscitation in cases of ventricular tachycardia (VT) when it is given as a 300-mg bolus via any intravenous access followed by an infusion if needed. In the acute state, it is

---

* There is wide debate on the best regimen for amiodarone use. For clarity, the suggestions of the *BNF* are presented but individual units may have different policies.

Table 28.1 Antiarrhythmic drugs. All class I drugs block the sodium channels in excitable tissues; sotalol is also a beta-blocker.

Class	Example	Effects	Indication
Ia	Disopyramide	Membrane depressant drugs, lengthen action potential	AF, SVT, VT
Ib	Lidocaine	Membrane depressant drugs, shorten action potential	VT/VF after MI
Ic	Flecainide	Membrane depressant drugs, no effect on action potential	VT/VF and SVT
II	Beta-blockers	Antisympathetic action	AF, PSVT
III	Amiodarone, sotalol	Prolong action potential without effect on sodium channels	AF, VT/VF, SVT
IV	Calcium-channel blockers	Reduce plateau phase of the action potential	PSVT

AF, atrial fibrillation; MI, myocardial infarction; PSVT, paroxysmal supraventricular tachycardia; SVT, supraventricular tachycardia; VF, ventricular fibrillation; VT, ventricular tachycardia.

generally accepted that 300 mg i.v. given over 10–15 min followed by 900 mg over the next 24 h gives high levels initially. After this, 600 mg/day orally in divided doses for 3–5 days provides a satisfactory steady state. Maintenance is usually 200–300 mg/day. Intravenous doses for maintenance are the same and given over 2–4 h.

The bolus can be given peripherally with a large volume flush. For the remainder, large veins should be used with a running flush or, preferably, central access. Oral loading for less acute indications can be given as 200 mg t.d.s. for 5 days followed by 200 mg b.d. for 5 days, then maintenance of 200–300 mg/day. The oral preparation is associated with slightly better rhythm control properties than the intravenous approach, which has a greater class IV (calcium–channel blocker) effect. The reason for this is unclear, but may be because of rapid increases in plasma levels.

Multiple loading episodes may be tried on the same patient, although the evidence for this is scant.

Amiodarone significantly increases the effects of warfarin and digoxin.

Amiodarone can cause severe myocardial depression and bradycardia (asystole) if given very rapidly. The intravenous bolus over 30 s method is reserved for cardiac arrest situations.

Sotalol

This class III drug has weak beta-blocking properties but can still induce bronchospasm in susceptible patients. Its main use is in the prophylaxis of supraventricular rhythm disturbances and the acute treatment of ventricular arrhythmia. The dosage is 80–640 mg/day in two divided doses. Intravenous preparations are not often used routinely.

The use of this drug with others can lead to further conduction abnormalities and may precipitate heart block. It should not be used with verapamil.

Flecainide

This is a potent drug used for atrial antiarrhythmic and junctional re-entry tachycardias. It is not commonly used for ventricular arrhythmias in the UK, although it does have a licence for this. Long-term use in patients with structural heart diseases or heart failure is associated with an increase in mortality. It is becoming the treatment of choice for the acute management of supraventricular tachycardia (SVT) in otherwise healthy young patients.

The intravenous dose is 2 mg/kg (maximum 150 mg) given over 10–30 min. If an infusion is needed, a dose of 1.5 mg/kg is given over 1 h followed by 100–250 micrograms/kg/h for 24 h (maximum 600 mg/24 h). The oral dose is 50–200 mg b.d.

Digoxin

Digoxin is a cardiac glycoside that inhibits the sodium–potassium adenosine triphosphatase. This increases intracellular sodium, which in turn inhibits the sodium–calcium exchanger and leads to an increase in intracellular calcium. Through this effect, digoxin increases myocardial contractility. It reduces conduction through the atrioventicular (AV) node via a poorly understood mechanism that probably partly involves enhancement of vagal tone. It is not really an antiarrhythmic as it does not cardiovert but, by slowing down conduction, may improve cardiac function.

Digoxin is predominantly used for the control of ventricular response to persistent atrial fibrillation (AF). It is less commonly used as a treatment for cardiac failure. Starting the drug depends on the precise indication (Table 28.2).

Oral digoxin is rapidly absorbed and is given in a once daily regimen for maintenance. The oral loading dose is 1250–1500 micrograms over 18 h and should be given at regular divided intervals. The maintenance dose is between 62.5 and 250 micrograms/day.

Digoxin can be given intravenously for emergency rate control. A range of protocols exists but, in essence, the loading dose is 1250 micrograms over 10–14 h. Traditionally, a bolus of 500 micrograms given over 30 min is followed by a further bolus of 500 micrograms 4–6 h later and then 250 micrograms 8–12 h after that. This allows for initially high plasma levels before decaying to a steady state. The last dose can be given orally and the maintenance dose is usually between 62.5 and 250 micrograms once daily as

Table 28.2 Protocols for starting treatment with digoxin.

Clinical urgency	Treatment
No urgency	Oral loading and maintenance
Rapid treatment	Intravenous or oral loading with oral maintenance
Urgent treatment	Intravenous loading and close review

before. At higher doses very careful drug level monitoring is needed. In the acute setting, if a rate reduction does not ensue after a full loading dose, further clinical and biochemical review is needed and electrical cardioversion may be indicated.

Digoxin is renally cleared and the dosage should be reduced in renal failure and in the elderly. The ventricular rate will help to guide loading and maintenance dose selection. Hypokalaemia enhances digoxin toxicity and plasma electrolytes should be corrected prior to its use and checked regularly thereafter. Digoxin should therefore be used with particular caution in patients on diuretics, which predispose to hypokalaemia. Such patients may need either to be switched to a potassium-sparing diuretic or given potassium supplements. Plasma levels do not routinely have to be measured, although if this is done then it should be performed 6 h after a dose. Digoxin will have additive effects, as with all rate controlling agents such as calcium-channel blockers and amiodarone.

Digoxin is contra-indicated in second- or intermittent third-degree heart block. It should not be used in patients who have aberrant accessory AV conduction pathways, such as Wolff–Parkinson–White syndrome.

A patient with a new cardiac arrhythmia on digoxin should have his/her plasma levels measured. Digoxin toxicity usually manifests as a bradycardia or heart block but patients may also present with other rhythms. Correcting any hypokalaemia will help in cases of digoxin toxicity. Digoxin-specific antibody can be used in specialized units for the treatment of toxicity.

> Digoxin will not cardiovert an aberrant rhythm but does allow rate control. This may be a satisfactory option in many cases of atrial fibrillation.

Adenosine

This drug is used for cardiac stress testing, to assess native pacemaker function and, most commonly, to cause transient AV nodal blockade and a suppression of sinoatrial (SA) node activity. This allows atrial activity to be defined and can cardiovert SVTs. It should not be used if accessory pathways are likely (as for digoxin, above). The drug has a half-life measured in seconds and can be given as an intravenous bolus. The initial dose should be 3 mg. If this is ineffective, after a couple of minutes, further doses of 6 mg and then 12 mg can be given. For safety, keep the line flushed with a running drip. The patient should be warned that he/she will experience flushing, tight chest and limb heaviness for a short period.

Role of magnesium and potassium

Reduced plasma levels of potassium are associated with rhythm disturbances and intravenous and oral replacement should be carried out to maintain plasma levels; 4–5 mmol/L may be required. Hypomagnesaemia may also be clinically significant; a bolus of magnesium sulphate (8–10 mmol) given over 10–15 min (and repeated if needed) may be useful in serious arrhythmias. The plasma levels of magnesium do not need to be measured before this dose. If there is a low magnesium plasma concentration, 70 mmol can be given as a slow infusion via a syringe driver over 24 h.

Beta-blockers and calcium-channel blockers have antiarrhythmic properties, which are considered in Chapter 26.

Atrial fibrillation and flutter

Atrial fibrillation and flutter are probably the arrhythmias most commonly encountered in the general setting. Risk factors include ischaemic heart disease, toxins including alcohol, acute metabolic stresses, especially postoperatively, and thyroid disease. AF is seen more commonly in the elderly population.

As a general rule, sinus rhythm is a better situation than any rhythm disturbance. Cardiac output is more stable and efficient and the risk of systemic emboli is less. In any presentation of rhythm problem, the urgency for regaining rate or rhythm control has to be established and this guides therapy; AF is no different.

If there is cardiovascular compromise caused by AF, rapid cardioversion or rate control is needed, whatever the aetiology of AF. This can be done with DC synchronous shocks (*in extremis* only), or a combination of agents for rate and rhythm.

In the postoperative patient, AF can result from many causes. Most often, this is transient and resolves with adequate correction of fluid and electrolytes. AF during sepsis from any source is difficult to cardiovert electrically for any length of time as the underlying problem remains. Chemical cardioversion may be useful and amiodarone has become the drug of choice,

unless the patient is otherwise healthy with a normal heart when flecainide can be considered. Often rate control is sufficient while the infection is treated. This can be done using intravenous digoxin in the compromised patient and oral digoxin otherwise. Make sure magnesium levels have been supplemented (8–10 mmol bolus) and potassium levels corrected (4–5 mmol/L).

Verapamil and beta-blockers are also used for rapid rate control in any compromising atrial tachyarrhythmia. This should be performed with close monitoring and in experienced hands because of the risk of myocardial depression.

Amiodarone and digoxin each potentiate the side-effects of the other and may hasten rate control if given together acutely.

Anticoagulation for rhythm disturbances

A wealth of clinical evidence exists regarding this issue [1–3]. New data are constantly being produced and it is beyond the scope of this book to discuss them in depth.

The principles guiding therapy and prescription are as follows.

1 Patients over 75 years at high risk of a stroke benefit from anticoagulation with dose-adjusted warfarin with respect to the incidence of stroke.

2 Patients under 75 years with few risk factors may benefit a little but not significantly more than if taking antiplatelet agents.

3 Patients under 65 years at low risk of stroke do not benefit from anticoagulation and should be offered aspirin.

The incidence of major bleeding is increased in the elderly. The risk of bleeding is greater if the INR is elevated above 4. Around 50% of patients at high risk of bleeding will have a major bleed within 2 years if anticoagulated [4]. The risks of bleeding are greater in those over 65 years; with a history of bleeding; stroke; or any of MI, renal impairment or diabetes. Anticoagulation with dose-adjusted warfarin should be offered to any patient at high risk of a stroke with moderate or low risk of a bleed. Antiplatelet agents should be given to the remainder. The INR should be closely monitored.

Having decided to anticoagulate, the need for acute INR control is less pressing and so a gradual loading regimen can be employed. One method is to carry out the baseline checks as normal and start 2 mg/day warfarin for 5 days and repeat INR. Doses can then be adjusted as normal.* This allows for out-patient or GP management.

Normal protocols for warfarinization can also be used if the patient is likely to be in hospital anyway.

AF can be precipitated by myocardial ischaemia and this should always be sought. Also, fast AF may result in ischaemia.

References

1 European Atrial Fibrillation Trial Study Group. Optimal oral anticoagulant therapy in patients with non-rheumatic atrial fibrillation and recent cerebral ischemia. *N Engl J Med* 1995; **333**: 5–10.

2 Atrial Fibrillation Investigators. The efficacy of aspirin in patients with atrial fibrillation: analysis of pooled data from three randomised trials. *Arch Intern Med* 1997; **157**: 1237–40.

3 Gage BF, Cardinalli AB, Albers GW, Owens DK. Cost-effectiveness of warfarin and aspirin for prophylaxis of stroke in patients with non-valvular atrial fibrillation. *J Am Med Assoc* 1995; **274**: 1839–45.

4 Beyth RJ, Quinn LM, Landefeld CS. Prospective evaluation of an index for predicting the risk of major bleeding in outpatients treated with warfarin. *Am J Med* 1998; **105**: 91–9.

---

* This method seems to be widely used effectively but with little published evidence.

29: **Airways disease**

Asthma and chronic obstructive pulmonary disease

Airways disease of any sort is a diagnosis that is often made without formal assessment. A trial of therapy is started and the patient soon has a label so that any worsening of symptoms is met with an increase in drug therapy rather than a review of diagnosis. The result is a patient with genuine cough or dyspnoea-type symptoms on maximal steroid and bronchodilator therapy which may not be appropriate.

There is no single test that is diagnostic for asthma or chronic obstructive pulmonary disease (COPD). Careful history and examination are important. When you encounter a patient who has a history of asthma or COPD and is on therapy, take time to establish when and how that diagnosis was made. Were formal reversibility studies carried out to beta-agonists and steroids? What is the report of the last chest X-ray? How are the prescribed medications actually being taken? What is the best PEFR?

Treatment

For both asthma and COPD, the patient should be strongly encouraged to give up smoking. Asthmatics should also be counselled, where appropriate, about the need to avoid allergen triggers. Most hospitals have a specialist respiratory nurse who is able to provide support for patients and ward staff alike. Use his/her expertise early in any admission and also for discharge follow-up.

Pharmacological treatments

Algorithms for the treatment of acute and chronic asthma exist in the *BNF*, as produced by the British Thoracic Society (BTS). These are based on guidelines that have appeared in journal form and will not be repeated here [1].

In general terms, patients should be taught the difference between drugs used for symptomatic relief, such as beta-agonists, and drugs used for prophylaxis, such as inhaled steroids. Compliance is important and is reinforced by patient education.

Drugs available

Beta$_2$-agonists

Beta-agonists, such as salbutamol or terbutaline, provide rapid and effective bronchodilatation. Some overlap beta$_1$ effects will result in tachycardia and tremor which may be quite severe. At the start of therapy, patients may receive occasional inhaled salbutamol. Regular therapy with short-acting agents is inappropriate. Long-acting agents are becoming increasingly useful and are usually given twice a day. They should be prescribed if there are more than just occasional symptoms and are best used in combination with inhaled steroids. They also come in a range of preparations of which the pressurized metered-dose inhaler (MDI) is the most common. They are not useful in the acute setting.

Oral preparations of beta-agonists are available and most often prescribed in the very elderly or those with difficulty in using the preferred inhalation route. The long-acting oral bambuterol (a prodrug of terbutaline) has a place in the therapy of predominantly nocturnal symptoms.

Intravenous salbutamol or terbutaline is used in acute severe asthma. If using intravenous salbutamol, make up 5 mg in 500 mL dextrose and give via any line. Start at 50 mL/h and titrate to response. Cardiac monitoring is needed. Continuous subcutaneous infusions of terbutaline are sometimes used in difficult to control asthma, although this route is not advised for most cases.

Antimuscarinic agents

Drugs in this category appear in the BTS treatment algorithms for acute asthma but are more effective in COPD. They usually start to work within 60 min and effects are seen up to 6 h later. These are prescribed in four times daily regimens. Very long-acting versions are as yet unavailable. There is less effect on the heart than with beta-agonists and this may be more useful when tachycardia is to be avoided. Combination versions with salbutamol exist *(Combivent)* and are useful as rescue therapy. At the time of writing, long-acting beta-agonists and antimuscarinic combinations were not widely available.

Theophyllines

This class of drug has a place in bronchospasm that is difficult to manage. They are given orally for maintenance therapy and by the intravenous route for severe exacerbations of disease. These drugs have a very narrow therapeutic index and it may be useful to measure plasma levels of the drug to ensure maximal therapeutic benefit. A level of 10–20 mg/L is normally the aim.

This is potentially a dangerous class of drug. Before starting intravenous treatment of acute severe asthma with aminophylline (500 micrograms/kg/h), it is important to check that the patient is not taking oral theophylline preparations. Overdose (or excessively fast intravenous treatment) is associated with vomiting, agitation, arrhythmias, hypokalaemia and convulsions. Theophylline preparations are not equivalent and provide a rare example of a drug that should be prescribed by brand (proprietary) name.

The half-life of theophyllines is increased in heart failure, cirrhosis and the elderly. It is also increased by cimetidine and the oral contraceptive pill. The half-life is reduced in smokers, heavy drinkers and by drugs including phenytoin and carbamazepine.

Corticosteroids

These drugs are very effective in asthma but much less effective in pure COPD. Indeed, it is useful to formally test for steroid effectiveness in COPD patients. There is little evidence that there is long-term benefit in this group but there may be some improvement in acute exacerbations. They act principally by reducing airway inflammation and oedema. The inhaled route is preferred as the systemic side-effects of steroids are reduced, but oral preparations are available for acute exacerbations and the intravenous route is used when this is not possible. Nebulized steroid solutions are also available.

Oral prednisolone may be useful in patients with exacerbations of asthma. This can be given for 7–10 days at 40 mg/day and stopped without much concern for adrenal suppression. In patients with poorer asthma control, however, sudden cessation of steroids may give rise to a relapse of symptoms. Longer prescriptions should be gradually stepped down at approximately 5–10 mg at a time every 5 days.

The side-effects in the elderly population can be very debilitating (e.g. osteoporosis-related fractures) and a reflex prescription of steroids should be avoided.

Combination long-acting beta-agonists and steroids are very useful. The prescription charge is as for a single agent and so this will dramatically reduce the costs for patients at discharge.

Mucolytics

There is good evidence that long-term use of mucolytics significantly reduces the frequency of exacerbations of COPD [2]. Mecysteine hydrochloride 100–200 mg t.d.s. orally is used. In some centres, nebulized N-acetylcysteine is used and local policy should be sought.

Leukotriene antagonists

These have an evolving role in the management of childhood asthma, especially in cases related to significant atopy. They are of questionable use in adults. They have no role in the management of an acute exacerbation.

Anxiolytics

In COPD and asthma, emotion and anxiety can make the symptoms of an acute event much worse. The helpless feeling of not being able to breathe must be very frightening. Along with any medication that is prescribed, reassurance in a calm environment is of great help. Regular anxiolysis with low sedation might be useful in elderly COPD patients. Paroxetine and trimipramine at low doses are good for this.

Routes and methods of delivery

Inhalation

This has the advantage of delivering the drug directly to its desired site of action. The drugs are delivered in a metered-dose fashion using a variety of proprietary devices or via a nebulizer chamber.

Pressure-activated metered-dose inhaler

This is by far the most commonly prescribed device. It delivers a set dose of drug when activated. Button-activated systems need good hand grip, strength and co-ordination with inspiration. This should be demonstrated to the patient and re-emphasizes the usefulness of the specialist nurse in this regard. The pressurized MDIs use environmentally friendly agents but many patients will be used to the chlorofluorocarbon (CFC)-driven versions which are now being withdrawn. These will 'taste' different and may lead to a compliance problem, especially in children.

Breath-actuated inhalers and dry powder inhalers

These formats, which require a high inspiratory flow rate to trigger the device, are useful in adults with poor technique in using button-activated systems, although they may still be unsuitable for children. Bioavailability is reduced with dry powder inhalers, so doses are usually doubled.

In most pressurized systems, the high-velocity stream may hit the back of the oropharynx so reducing the amount that enters the lungs. This is probably happening if the patient can 'taste' the drug. A large volume spacer is a device that slows down the aerosol particle velocity and allows the propellant to evaporate, so aiding inhalation of the active agent. The most efficient have a large volume with one-way valves.

It is good practice to prescribe a spacer device to anyone with less than perfect technique, which, in practice, is most people. The pharmacy will issue one most appropriate to the MDI you have chosen.

Nebulizers

A nebulizer is a chamber in which a volume of active drug sits in solution. The solution is converted into an aerosol by high flow gas or ultrasonically. The type of nebulizer, rate of gas flow or ultrasound setting and properties of the drug in question will determine the re-

sultant particle size and hence the amount of drug that reaches the lung.

Bronchodilators, steroids and some antibiotics can be nebulized. At best, 30% of the drug will end up in the lung but most commonly it is less than 10%. The indications for nebulizer use are therefore limited and include the following.

1 Delivery of drug to a patient with an acute exacerbation of asthma or COPD.
2 Delivery of drug to a patient with drug-responsive disease needing high doses.
3 Delivery of drug to a patient with poor technique with the above methods.

Home nebulizers usually use a portable air compressor to drive the system. These are noisy but effective. Oxygen cylinders for use in the community cannot generate the necessary high flow rates needed (around 6 L/min). In hospital, air cylinders, and preferably oxygen, are easily available and should be used instead. Increased vigilance is needed in COPD patients who are CO_2 retainers but this does not normally require avoidance of oxygen-driven nebulizers.

Other routes

Tablets and syrups are available as are solutions for intravenous or subcutaneous infusions.

Common prescribing concerns

1 *Beta-blockers and beta-agonists prescribed together.* Occasionally, the need for beta-blockade outweighs some resultant wheeze and highly cardioselective

agents can be used, but this should be carried out with specialist advice, a definite long-term plan and regular PEFR checks.

2 *As required salmeterol.* This is a long-acting beta-agonist and it makes little sense giving it at irregular intervals.

3 *Salbutamol inhaler six times a day.* This should be replaced with increased doses of long-acting agent with some salbutamol available on an 'as required' basis.

4 *Oral steroids and inhaled steroids at the same time.* In the acute setting, this is unnecessary. When inhaled steroids are being reintroduced, the oral preparation still needs to be reduced in a stepwise fashion.

5 *NSAIDs and bronchodilators.* A percentage of the asthmatic population may become more symptomatic with concurrent NSAID therapy. In a few cases, acute bronchospasm may be induced. This is not a reason to avoid NSAIDs in asthmatics automatically, merely to be more vigilant with history-taking, clinical judgement and PEFR charts. However, if significant deterioration is seen, this should be listed in the 'sensitivities section' of the chart and the patient warned accordingly.

6 *Failure to change to the patient's usual delivery system on leaving hospital.* It is clearly essential to do this and review technique.

References

1 British Thoracic Society and others. Guidelines on the management of asthma. *Thorax* 1997; **52**: S1–S21.

2 Poole PJ, Black PN. Mucolytic agents for chronic bronchitis or chronic obstructive pulmonary disease. *Cochrane Database Syst Rev* 2000; **2**: CD001287.

30: **Oxygen therapy**

Oxygen therapy can be given to improve oxygenation for a range of clinical benefits from improving wound healing to decreasing confusion. In the majority of patients, the exact amount of oxygen delivered is not important. Furthermore, although there is some merit in maximizing oxygen availability in the acute setting, in general, titrating the supply of oxygen to the arterial pressure of oxygen (Pao_2) and pulse oximetry is preferred. However, in cases of type 2 respiratory failure, oxygen delivery must be much more accurately undertaken and closely monitored.

Determinants of oxygen delivery

The fraction of inspired oxygen (Fio_2) will depend upon the following.
1 Flow of oxygen. If the flow of oxygen is much less than the peak inspiratory flow rate, then maximum oxygen delivery is compromised.
2 Presence or absence of any reservoir.
3 Interface between patient and supply (i.e. mask, nasal cannulae, oxygen tent, etc.).

Face masks and nasal cannulae

An oxygen mask is adequate for most cases, with the simple Hudson mask being perhaps the most commonly used. Fio_2 from this system is variable, however, and some patients find such masks claustrophobic. Nasal cannulae are an alternative to the Hudson mask and may be better tolerated by the patient, causing less interference with eating, drinking and speaking. A drawback is that they may cause nasopharyngeal irritation or ulceration.

It is difficult to be certain what Fio_2 is being delivered with this system. From 24 to 40% may be achieved. Nasal cannulae set to $2\,L/min$ flow rate may produce an Fio_2 of approximately 30% with proper use. This system is adequate when therapy can be titrated to pulse oximetry values and where there is little danger of blunting respiratory drive.

Fixed performance masks

Fixed performance systems are better when accurate provision of oxygen is needed. These work on the principle of high-flow oxygen enrichment. A Venturi valve attached to a mask allows high-flow oxygen to be delivered to the patient. Its passage through the valve entrains air at a fixed rate. This combined flow rate is so high (up to $40\,L/min$) that the expired (alveolar) air cannot accumulate and the peak inspiratory flow rate is easily met. The O_2 flow rate and the properties of the valve thus determine the Fio_2. Most common valves provide an Fio_2 of 24, 28, 32 or 45%. Variations on this allow for humidification and can provide up to 60%; this is seen with the *Respiflow*.

Reservoirs

Higher concentrations of $F\text{io}_2$ can be achieved with a non-rebreathing mask and reservoir. This consists of a 1-L reservoir bag, a face mask and high-flow oxygen. The bag acts as a reservoir of pure O_2 and, when the patient inhales, over 90% of it will be oxygen, allowing for the slight rebreathing and entrainment of air that are inevitable with a standard mask.

An $F\text{io}_2$ of 100% will only be achieved using formal airway support or a tight-fitting non-invasive mask. Humidification should be considered with any device if prolonged use of oxygen therapy is envisaged or there is productive lung disease.

Respiratory failure

In acute or acute on chronic hypoxia, oxygen therapy should not be withheld for fear of diminishing respiratory drive. It is the hypoxia that kills the patient, so just provide increased vigilance. Your prescription should define the $F\text{io}_2$ or flow rate, method of delivery, humidification, target range of pulse oximetry values and duration of therapy. For example, a prescription might read, 'Continuous oxygen via a 45% Venturi mask and valve: target saturations of 100%'.

Type 1 respiratory failure

This is defined as hypoxia ($Pa\text{o}_2$ less than 8 kPa or 60 mmHg) without hypercapnia. The aim of therapy is to improve oxygenation and so the pulse oximetry or arterial saturations should be titrated to response. A variable system may be adequate here.

Type 2 respiratory failure

This is defined as hypoxia with hypercapnia ($Pa\text{co}_2$ more than 7 kPa or 55 mmHg). Here the aim is to provide safe but not normal levels of oxygenation. A $Pa\text{o}_2$ around 8 kPa or saturations of over 85% may well be acceptable. Prescribe the lowest concentration of oxygen to achieve this level of oxygenation. This requires a fixed performance system although once a steady state has been reached low-flow nasal cannulae can be used in chronic cases.

Discharge prescriptions for oxygen

There is an agreement that oxygen prescriptions are provided by GPs autonomously or under guidance from hospital colleagues. As in hospital, the oxygen can be on an 'as-required' basis to cover times of exertion and to manage short acute episodes. This is done through liquid oxygen cylinders that have a number of preset flow rates.

For some, long-term therapy is needed. This must be initiated following an assessment in hospital (details in Section 3.6 of the *BNF*) [1]. The hospital discharge script should have the O_2 therapy noted to provide a record, but should state that it is not to be dispensed by the pharmacy.

Reference

1 Rees PJ, Dudley F. ABC of oxygen: provision of oxygen at home. *Br Med J* 1998; **317**: 935–8.

31: **Musculoskeletal drugs**

Treatment of joint and muscle disease forms a significant part of daily prescribing. These can be dealt with as pain relief, other symptom control and disease modification. Much of these are covered elsewhere in this book.

Osteoarthritis

This is degenerative joint disease that can also manifest as soft tissue inflammation, muscle atrophy and deformity. Pain relief follows the analgesic ladder and regularly taken paracetamol and low-dose NSAIDs are usually sufficient. Corticosteroids injected into the joint space may also provide some temporary relief. Hyaluronic acid and derivatives can help slow the degenerative process over a period of months with improved function but may exacerbate inflammation in the early stages. Muscle relaxants and antispasmodics can help also. Use of long-term NSAIDs is associated with a wealth of adverse effects, principally peptic ulceration, so prophylaxis for this should be considered.

Non-drug therapy such as weight loss and exercise should be encouraged.

Gout

NSAIDs, colchicine and allopurinol are the drugs used, and treatment should be addressed by reducing the uric acid load

with weight reduction, proper diet and attention to prescriptions (thiazides can exacerbate gout).

In the acute setting, allopurinol may exacerbate symptoms. High-dose oral NSAIDs can be used, but with regard for renal and gastric function. Once the pain is under control, allopurinol can be started.

Colchicine

Colchicine is only as effective as NSAIDs but has a role when the patient is on diuretics (as it has less fluid-retaining effects) or anticoagulants. Toxic levels are soon reached and dosing should be stopped when severe gastrointestinal upset is seen. A dose of 1 mg is given immediately followed by 500 micrograms every 2 h until relief is obtained. The maximum dosage is 6 mg within 3 days.

Allopurinol

This can be started after an estimate of uric acid levels has been made and a clinical need established. The dose is initially 100 mg o.d., rising to a maintenance of 900 mg/day in divided doses depending on uric acid levels. A rash may be seen at the start of therapy; if so, withdraw at once as marked hypersensitivity-type reactions are seen. One month of administration of colchicine (500 micrograms t.d.s. orally) or NSAIDs should be given as prophylaxis against acute attacks of gout that may be precipitated by treatment. The patient must be well hydrated.

Allopurinol forms a part of chemo- and radiotherapy regimens as prophylaxis.

Rheumatoid disease

This presents in a wide range of ways. Simple analgesics for joint and muscle pain are used but NSAIDs form the mainstay of therapy. COX-2 inhibitors are alternatives. Pain modification therapy with low-dose amitriptyline (25 mg) is also used widely. Intra-articular steroid injections are also used.

As for osteoarthritis, muscle spasm and soft tissue inflammation can be treated symptomatically using topical NSAIDs, which may be massaged onto the affected part of the body.

Disease modification antirheumatic drugs

Gold, penicillamine, antimalarials and immunosuppressants

These work through a range of mechanisms to alter the inflammatory process. Newer immunosuppressant agents are becoming available, including agents that target very specific points on the inflammatory cascade, such as tumour necrosis factor. These drugs should be initiated and maintained by specialists in a hospital setting.

A patient on one disease modification antirheumatic drug (DMARD) with little improvement should be tried on another, as responses vary greatly. A patient admitted on a DMARD with a flare of arthritis or indeed another pathology needs careful assessment. Most drugs of this type can produce blood dyscrasias. There should be caution for use in renal or liver failure. Contact the local rheumatology service for advice at the time of admission.

Methotrexate is associated with pulmonary toxicity and its plasma levels are enhanced by the concurrent use of aspirin and other NSAIDs. The antifolate effects are enhanced by antibiotics that target the same pathway, such as trimethoprim. Folic acid 5 mg o.d. can be taken or folinic acid in acute toxicity.

Azathioprine effects are enhanced with allopurinol and the dosage should be reduced when used together. With cyclosporin the side-effect and interaction profile is extensive. Of the more common, renal failure is seen, NSAID-induced nephrotoxicity is enhanced and cyclosporin levels are increased by diltiazem, grapefruit juice and H_2-receptor blockers.

32: **Movement disorders and epilepsy**

Patients with movement disorders tend to display the best compliance with their medications. Patients will have adapted their lifestyle and the times of medication to maximize their function. They may also be quite reliant upon specific brands. Both may be disrupted on arrival at hospital, so ask patients to bring in their own medication and arrange for them to self-medicate in hospital.

Muscle spasms and nocturnal cramps

Quinine at 200–300 mg *nocte* orally may provide some relief from nocturnal leg cramps. The effects are rarely apparent before a few weeks of therapy and, even then, there may only be a marginal decrease in the frequency of symptoms. There is an impressive side-effect profile and a danger of precipitating arrhythmias. The digoxin dosage needs to be reduced.

Chronic muscle spasm and contractures can be helped with centrally acting agents that reduce muscle tone. They are best used in combination with physiotherapy. If a patient is mobilizing and weight bearing, loss of tone can further worsen function and so these drugs should be given with regular review. Diazepam can be used in the acute setting, with analgesics to help with painful spasms. Its principal benefits are the

multiplicity of routes of administration and the relative short-acting effects.

Baclofen acts at the spinal level, but is also sedating and can precipitate convulsions and muscle pain. Dosage is by the oral route, starting at 15 mg/day in divided doses to a maximum of 100 mg. In prolonged use, withdrawal must be slow. Often NSAIDs are used at the same time and there may be reduced excretion of baclofen as a result.

Epilepsy

Most antiseizure medications for long-term use have a distinct therapeutic window with increasing side-effects at higher levels. Regular monitoring of levels is important (see Chapter 5). Monotherapy is still the preferred method and, if control is poor, the other available agents should be tried in sequence. Combination of agents may provide better control but will potentiate side-effects and increase toxic symptoms. Tricyclic antidepressants reduce the effects of anticonvulsants.

The peak plasma values determine the side-effect profile and so the regimen should be designed to have as few peaks and troughs as possible. The anticonvulsants used commonly affect gamma-aminobutyric acid (GABA) transmission, either by enhancement of effect or increased release.

The dosage and special precautions list is exhaustive in the *BNF*. All the drugs can be given via a nasogastric tube and carbamazepine has a rectal preparation with a maximum dosage of 1 g/day in divided doses.

In general, hepatic enzyme inducers will reduce efficacy and other anticonvulsants will augment activity.

Pregnancy and breast-feeding

In pregnancy, plasma levels may fall a little. There is a risk of teratogenicity with neural tube defects, but conventional management is to continue therapy as the risks to mother and fetus are greater if seizures are uncontrolled. All women who may become pregnant should be counselled prior to starting therapy. Folate supplements should be prescribed before and during pregnancy. Vitamin K should be offered to the mother before delivery, and also to the neonate if using carbamazepine or phenytoin as there is an increased risk of bleeding.

Breast-feeding does not carry more significant risk with standard regimens of conventional agents. However, it should be avoided with gabapentin and the manufacturers advise avoidance with phenytoin, although the levels are likely to be very small.

Phenytoin

Phenytoin is used in the acute setting for control of seizures before definitive therapy can be instituted. It is also used as maintenance therapy for all forms of epilepsy, but is increasingly being superseded as it has a narrow therapeutic window and zero order kinetics. Close cardiac monitoring is needed during infusions. The plasma target range is 40–80 µmol/L.

Carbamazepine

Carbamazepine is used in most forms of epilepsy, especially complex partial seizures. The dose–response is linear and there is a wider therapeutic window than with phenytoin. It is given in a twice daily regimen and plasma levels can be measured at the trough, aiming for 20–50 µmol/L. It also comes as a rectal preparation, which is useful if a patient cannot eat for any reason. This route should only be used for a maximum of 7 days and there is a dosing change: 125 mg given p.r.n. may be considered equivalent to 100 mg given daily. Controlled release preparations have lesser side-effects as the peak levels are lower.

Sodium valproate

Sodium valproate has a similar efficacy to carbamazepine and phenytoin. The effects do not appear to be related to plasma concentration and so routine monitoring in this case is not needed. Liver function is affected transiently in many cases at the start of therapy but this can persist and worsen, so liver function tests should be monitored while the patient is becoming established on the drug and at regular intervals thereafter.

Other drugs

Lamotrigine can be used as monotherapy but more often as adjuvant to another agent, usually sodium valproate. The dosage is different depending on the combination chosen and care should be taken on switching regimens. If a patient attends on a particular combination, try to stay on it. Sudden increases in dosage are associated with severe hypersensitivity reactions. If the patient has been off the drug for more than 1 week, it should be reintroduced at low doses once more.

Gabapentin is used as adjuvant therapy and for neuropathic pain.

Status epilepticus

This is a medical emergency and it is important to control the seizure rapidly. Oxygen should be given via a face mask. Intravenous lorazepam is the agent of choice in the acute setting. The initial dose is 4 mg i.v. with close monitoring and the availability of resuscitation equipment. The intramuscular and rectal routes are generally too slow to be effective but, in the absence of other access, a solution of diazepam can be given rectally at a maximum dose of 0.5 mg/kg in adults. The rectal tubes come in prefilled 2.5-, 5- and 10-mg doses, which all look quite similar.

The liberal use of benzodiazepines may well terminate the seizure but can also lead to prolonged coma in the post-ictal phase. If rectal or intramuscular drugs have been used, there may be a delay in clinical effect and additive effect. Keep a careful record of what was given, via which route and observe the patient appropriately. Giving reversal agents in this setting is not advised, as further seizures may well occur.

If the seizures persist, airway support and barbiturate anaesthesia may be needed. This will require the presence of specialist staff. It is prudent to check blood sugars and to check whether other precipitants such as drug abuse or overdose should take place at the same time.

Parkinsonian symptoms

The mainstay of pharmacological therapy in Parkinson's disease is dopamine replacement therapy. This is best suited to the idiopathic form, but has some limited role in parkinsonism of other aetiologies. It is inappropriate to commence therapy in newly suspected cases until a detailed clinical examination has been made as diagnosis after therapy has started can be difficult. The multidisciplinary approach is vital here and physiotherapists and occupational therapists should be involved in care. This is a specialist subject and is only covered briefly here.

Common therapies

Antimuscarinic drugs are used in the treatment of mild extrapyramidal symptoms (of any aetiology), especially if these are induced by the use of antipsychotics. If there is intercurrent depression or anxiety, the weak anticholinergic effects of the tricyclic agents, such as amitriptyline, may be useful (50–75 mg amitriptyline o.d. *nocte*).

Most dopamine replacement is in combination with inhibitors to the extracerebral dopa-decarboxylase. These are benserazide (*Madopar*) or carbidopa (*Sinemet*). This allows for smaller doses of dopamine to be used and hence fewer systemic side-effects. The prescription should indicate the doses of both elements and also the preferred brand name. Controlled release (CR) preparations can be substituted for more frequent dosage once good control has been achieved with short-acting agents. A combination of normal and CR formulations is often used. Examples are as follows.

• Co-beneldopa 50/200 is made up of 50 mg benserazide and 200 mg levodopa. It is prescribed as *Madopar 250*.

• Co-careldopa 12.5/50 is made up of 12.5 mg carbidopa and 50 mg levodopa and was sold as *Sinemet LS* but is now called *Sinemet-62.5*.

There is no need to give more than 75 mg/day carbidopa in any preparation as this produces maximal inhibition of dopa-decarboxylase. Also, there is no merit in combining dopa-decarboxylase inhibitors. Prescriptions should take this into account. *Madopar* can be given as a dispersible tablet and *Sinemet* can be crushed if needed (not the CR versions). This helps with administration through a nasogastric tube or similar. If a patient is established on CR preparations, and cannot take these for any reason, switch to a standard form with a slight reduction in dosage over the 24-h period.

Other therapies

• Selegiline is an MAO-B inhibitor. It has a role in early management and again in combination with levodopa to reduce end of dose symptoms. There is a reported overall increase in mortality with this combination. A patient stable on this therapy should not be withdrawn from it as this may precipitate worse symptoms.

• Bromocriptine is a dopamine receptor agonist and, together with the other ergot derivatives cabergoline and pergolide, it can help in the later stages of the disease. It has no role in drug-mediated extrapyramidal effects. There is a risk of pulmonary and retroperitoneal fibrosis and the CSM has suggested baseline erythrocyte sedimentation rate and chest X-ray prior to therapy. There is little increased benefit over levodopa therapy.

• Apomorphine. When therapy becomes difficult and there are marked symptoms, a continuous subcutaneous infusion of apomorphine can be used. This should only be initiated in hospital with specialist supervision (guidelines for this are in Section 4.9.1 of the *BNF*). If a patient is admitted to hospital on an apomorphine infusion or regular subcutaneous injections, these should be continued; the aim would be to reintroduce conventional therapy when possible.

Problems with therapy

As with all centrally stimulating drugs, antiparkinsonian medicines can lead to hallucinations and psychoses. High doses can cause an increase in involuntary movements. If side-effects are too great, especially at night time, a reduced dosage may be appropriate with a pragmatic acceptance of reduced nocturnal mobility.

Debilitating visual hallucinations and neuropsychiatric events should prompt a full review of medications and also a review of the diagnosis. A number of disease processes have extrapyramidal features also.

The most important rules for prescribing antiparkinsonian medications to an established patient are:

1 Do not change any drugs or doses without first discussing it with the patient and carers. Any unexpected change in symptoms can be very distressing.

2 Provide the antiparkinsonian medications at the times most suitable and

familiar to the patient. This may differ from standard drug rounds.

Drug-induced movement disorders

Tardive dyskinesia

This is the involuntary chewing and grimacing secondary to long-term antipsychotic use. The earliest sign is tongue smacking. It is more common in the elderly and usually responds to cessation of therapy. It can take months to settle down, however, and in some cases it never does. There is no really effective drug therapy.

Extrapyramidal symptoms and dystonias

These can be caused by antipsychotics and dopamine antagonists and may respond to antimuscarinic therapy. The individual responses to the various agents are wide and failure of one should prompt use of another. Common agents are procyclidine and benzatropine. These should be initially prescribed for the evening and at low doses and titrated up to the desired response. The dosage of procyclidine is from 2.5 mg o.d. to 30 mg/day in divided doses. Benzatropine can be given intravenously for emergency management of dystonias. A dose of 1–2 mg is given and repeated after 30 min if there is no resolution. This is preferable to using benzhexol (trihexyphenidyl) as benzatropine is more sedating and this feature is likely to be useful in this setting. There is no merit in prophylactic prescription of this drug class.

Do not rapidly stop antipsychotic use as the unmasked condition may be much more troublesome.

Tremor

This can be caused by overstimulation with thyroxine, beta-agonists or as a part of a withdrawal reaction. The first intervention is to examine the drug chart for likely causes. Benign essential tremor can also occur with no obvious precipitant. Usually, no therapy is needed but the antiepileptic drug primidone can be tried at very low doses (50 mg o.d.) in the morning. Beta-blockers may also be useful.

33: **Altered conscious level and stroke**

A deteriorating conscious level is often associated with altered oropharyngeal reflexes and hence safety of swallowing and protection of the airway may be an issue. There may be an antecedent systemic upset or, more often, a primary neurological event. The cause of the altered conscious level needs to be identified and any emergency procedures carried out. Once the cause is more established, routine and specialist drugs can be considered. If swallow function is questionable, oral medications are usually withheld or given via an enteral feeding tube, such as a nasogastric tube. This does not automatically protect the airway from aspiration as regurgitation is still possible.

Iatrogenic coma/reduced conscious level

Apart from drugs used directly in anaesthesia, the most common causes of drug-induced coma are opiate and benzodiazepine overdose. The use of reversal agents is covered in the relevant chapters. Hypoglycaemia is another very important cause.

A single bolus of reversal agent may identify the mechanism of the altered conscious level, but may not be adequately therapeutic. Do not just assume that a drug-induced coma has been adequa-

tely reversed. The patient must be observed regularly and further therapy given as needed. A patient might demand to self-discharge after a trial of reversal agent. This is to be discouraged until you are confident that reversal is complete and sustained.

Persistent reduced conscious level

The principles of prescribing should be directed to acute therapy depending on diagnosis, nutrition (preferably via the enteral route), normal medications if they are still appropriate, prophylaxis against DVT, infection, sores and contractures.

Stroke

The debate continues as to the best management of a stroke. There is some consensus that control of blood pressure, protection against secondary events, supportive therapy, nutrition and physiotherapy help in early improvement and probably in overall mortality [1].

Prescribing in stroke should take into account the limitations of oral intake because of an unsafe swallow, ease of administration, likely compliance at home and exaggerated side-effect profile. There may be a local stroke unit policy or protocol to follow that identifies initial therapeutic objectives and also limitations. Be guided by these.

141

In the initial stage, give adequate fluid intravenously and ensure tight glycaemic control using a sliding scale insulin regimen. Antiplatelet agents are advised in the acute setting for most strokes, unless there is sufficient evidence of a severe bleed or established coagulopathy (patient on warfarin). Early placement of a nasogastric tube facilitates the giving of normal medications. Until regular feeding is established, H_2-antagonists (or proton-pump inhibitor if there is a history of gastrointestinal bleed) should be given. Compression stockings should usually be fitted and full length ones should be used as soon as practicable. Check peripheral circulation first.

There is no indication for prophylactic antiepileptic use even in intracerebral bleeds. Cardiac dysrhythmias may have contributed to the stroke and this should be investigated further, but there is little evidence that an acute cardioversion improves early mortality or morbidity unless there is cardiovascular compromise.

Autoregulation is compromised following any cerebral insult and so blood pressure should not be aggressively treated without a complete diagnosis. Normal antihypertensive drugs can be restarted after approximately 48 h. Recent trial data promote the global use of statins in secondary prevention. These should be started acutely. However, this advice is not yet fully accepted. Full anticoagulation is not advised in most acute settings as even occlusive strokes can have further haemorrhagic transformation. Subcutaneous prophylactic heparin can be used.

Reference

1 Royal College of Physicans. *National Clinical Guidelines for Stroke, prepared by the Intercollegiate Working Party for Stroke, 1999.* Royal College of Physicians, June 2002.

34: **Constipation, diarrhoea and bowel disease**

Constipation

Constipation may be caused by a variety of disorders and these causes should be sought and treated. In all patients, general education about regular high-fibre diet with plenty of fluids should be advised.

Always be wary of the patient with obstruction. Clinical and radiological examinations should identify these patients before the inappropriate prescription of laxatives. Postoperative ileus is also common, even in patients who have not had abdominal surgery.

There are a number of drugs that are associated with constipation. These include opiates, tricyclic antidepressants, anticholinergic drugs, ferrous sulphate and calcium-channel blockers. In selected cases, such as opiate use, it is worth considering whether prophylactic laxatives should be prescribed.

Laxatives

There are a very large number of laxatives, which can be considered in categories according to their mechanism of action.

Bulk forming agents

These are hydrophilic compounds that act by absorbing water and increasing stool bulk. The effects of this are a stim-ulation of gut motility and rectal reflexes that promote defecation. These drugs are useful in patients with idiopathic constipation, diverticular disease, stomas, haemorrhoids and anal fissure. Patients should be advised to drink plenty of water with these preparations and warned that they may experience increased flatulence. Their mechanism of action means that they should be avoided in patients with adhesions, strictures and scleroderma. *Fybogel 150* can be made up in a small amount of water and taken twice a day.

Faecal softeners and lubricants

These act by softening the stool and lubricating the motion. They are commonly given either as enemas or suppositories. They are useful therapies for constipation associated with adhesions or strictures and for patients with a 'fear of defecation' brought on by anal fissure or haemorrhoids.

Osmotic laxatives

These act by retaining fluid in the stool by osmosis. Adequate fluid intake is required. These types of preparations may be taken orally or as enemas. Lactulose is a semisynthetic osmotic laxative that is not absorbed from the gastrointestinal tract. The resultant low faecal pH, which inhibits ammonia-producing bacteria, makes this particularly suitable for use in hepatic encephalopathy. Give lactulose 15–30 mL b.d. initially. In liver disease, give 30–50 mL b.d.

Stimulant laxatives

Stimulant laxatives, such as *Senokot*, increase intestinal motility. They may cause abdominal cramp-like pains. They should not be used in patients with obstruction. This is a commonly abused class of drugs and chronic use may result in colonic atony. Versions are available in oral or suppository form. The dosage is *Senokot* (7.5 mg) 2–4 tablets given at night for 3–5 days.

Co-danthramer is a potent laxative, but it has been shown to be teratogenic in rodents after prolonged exposure and so its use is limited to the terminal care setting.

Diarrhoea

Diarrhoea is a common problem and can have many causes. Consider the underlying cause of the problem. In patients coming from home, it is important to consider infective diarrhoea, inflammatory bowel disease, subtotal intestinal obstruction, faecal impaction with overflow diarrhoea or intra-abdominal disease such as abscess.

Another important cause of diarrhoea in patients who have recently had antibiotics (particularly clindamycin, although any antibiotic may be responsible) is pseudomembranous colitis. This is best treated with metronidazole 400 mg t.d.s. orally or vancomycin 125 mg q.d.s. orally, depending on local policy. However, generally gastroenteritis should not be treated with antibiotics.

Exceptions are *Campylobacter*, *Salmonella* and typhoid fever that can all be treated with ciprofloxacin.

Treatment

This should be directed towards the underlying cause. Resuscitation of the patient with oral or intravenous rehydration is very important alongside electrolyte correction.

Antidiarrhoeal medications

These can be used in simple diarrhoea in adults but should not be used in children. They can also be usefully used in patients with high-output stomas to thicken and decrease output. In patients with mild symptoms of incontinence, some improvement may be seen by hardening stool consistency.

Codeine phosphate

This is the antidiarrhoeal preferred by many clinicians. It should not be used in acute conditions, such as ulcerative colitis and pseudomembranous colitis. The usual dose is 15–60 mg q.d.s. orally titrated against symptoms.

Loperamide

This should be avoided in acute ulcerative colitis and pseudomembranous colitis. The usual starting dose is 4 mg followed by 2 mg after each loose stool up to a maximum of 16 mg/day.

Inflammatory bowel disease

Drugs involved in this debilitating spectrum of disorders are described but not explored in more detail. Their use should be directed by specialists.

Aminosalicylates

These are useful drugs for the treatment of relapse but their main use is for maintenance of remission. Sulfasalazine comprises 5-aminosalicylic acid and sulfapyridine. The sulfapyridine acts only as the carrier molecule, and is cleaved from the active component of the drug by the colonic flora. Many of the adverse effects of the drug are related to the sulfapyridine component of the drug. These are avoided in some of the newer aminosalicylates, including mesalazine, balsalazide and olsalazine [1].

Blood disorders can occur with any of this class of drugs. Patients should be warned that they should seek medical help if they develop unexplained bleeding, bruising, purpura, sore throat or fever. There is also a small but definite incidence of renal impairment or failure in patients taking these drugs. Renal function should be monitored and it has recently been suggested that this should be carried out every month for the first 3 months, every 3 months for 1 year and then annually [2]. Other side-effects include reversible oligospermia, diarrhoea, nausea, rash, headache and pancreatitis.

Corticosteroids

For disease localized to the rectum or distal colitis, local applications of steroids in the form of suppositories or enemas may be appropriate. For patients with more refractory disease or acute severe problems, these might be given orally or parenterally. Budesonide is an alternative steroid with a lower incidence of systemic side-effects.

Ulcerative colitis

Maintenance of remission in ulcerative colitis

Aminosalicylates are important in the maintenance of remission in ulcerative colitis. For distal colitis and proctitis, rectal preparations in the form of enemas or suppositories may be useful. A number of patients are intolerant to aminosalicylate drugs. In such patients, maintenance steroids are avoided as much as possible. In this regard, immunosuppressive drugs such as azathioprine may be helpful as steroid-sparing agents to maintain remission.

There is little evidence for the use of elemental diets in ulcerative colitis.

Treatment of severe acute ulcerative colitis or relapse

Steroids (orally or rectally) may be useful in disease flares that manifest as an increase in stool frequency without systemic illness. However, in more severe disease, in-patient treatment is required, with close liaison with the surgical team. Patients should be kept nil by mouth, with intravenous rehydration. Patients should be closely monitored with regular clinical examination, daily abdominal X-rays and daily blood tests, including inflammatory markers. Patients should be started on 100 mg hydrocortisone q.d.s. i.v. with twice daily steroid foam enemas. There is also interest in the use of cyclosporin in acute colitis.

If the patient settles, he/she can normally be switched to prednisolone 40 mg o.d. orally for 6 weeks, after which the dosage can be slowly decreased. An aminosalicylate should also be started. If the patient fails to settle, then surgical intervention may be necessary.

Crohn's disease

Maintenance of remission

Aminosalicylates may again be helpful for maintaining remission in Crohn's disease, although the evidence in this condition is less compelling. Corticosteroids are an option although, again, their use for maintenance treatment should be minimized. Immunosuppressants may be used as steroid-sparing agents.

Treatment of acute flares of disease

Steroids may be useful in the treatment of acute flares of the disease. Although there is little general evidence for the efficacy of antibiotics in inflammatory bowel disease, metronidazole is often used in perianal active Crohn's disease. Antibiotics can also be useful in the treatment of localized perforation and fistulas associated with sepsis.

Infliximab is a chimeric monoclonal antibody that has been introduced as a treatment for Crohn's disease resistant to steroids and immunosuppressants. It is particularly efficacious as a therapy for perianal fistulas. It is a specialist treatment that should only be started in an appropriate centre.

References

1 Ransford RA, Langman MJ. Sulphasalazine and mesalazine: serious adverse reactions re-evaluated on the basis of suspected adverse reaction reports to the Committee on Safety of Medicines. *Gut* 2002; **51**: 536–9.

2 Corrigan G, Stevens PE. Review article: interstitial nephritis associated with the use of mesalazine in inflammatory bowel disease. *Aliment Pharmacol Ther* 2000; **14**: 1–6.

35: **Nausea and vomiting**

Nausea and vomiting are very common throughout the hospital population. The centre for emesis lies in the lateral reticular formation and can be triggered by the chemoreceptor trigger zone on the floor of the fourth ventricle. Some of the causes of nausea and vomiting are listed in Table 35.1. Identifying the cause or stimulus of the symptom is crucially important as it is often more appropriate to treat the underlying cause rather than the nausea or vomiting itself.

Nausea or vomiting may limit the oral intake of fluid, nutrition or medications, compromising recovery. Elderly patients or those with significant concurrent disease are at greater risk. Medications that have been marked as given on the chart may not have been absorbed and so alternative routes of administration should be considered. Nutrition is often forgotten in such cases, so involve the ward dietitian early. Intravenous fluids are a simple intervention that can prevent the situation from deteriorating.

Consider if nausea is expected given the underlying disease; it may be necessary to chart medications regularly. Oral antiemetics can be useful but the actively vomiting patient needs intravenous administration. Intramuscular and rectal preparations can be used but it is worth securing intravenous access for fluid replacement.

Types of antiemetic

The antiemetic drug list includes a heterogeneous group of drug classes. Antiemetics can be used independently or in concert but can also antagonize each other.

Phenothiazines (e.g. prochlorperazine)

These are dopamine antagonists that act centrally. They are particularly useful in drug-induced symptoms (cytotoxic, opioid and general anaesthesia) and as an adjunct to mechanical decompression. The main side-effects are extrapyramidal motor problems but there is also a weak antimuscarinic effect, which may cause dry mouth and blurring of vision. Sedation can also be seen.

Start 20 mg orally, then continue at 10 mg every 2 h if needed: 12.5 mg i.m. or 25 mg p.r.n.

Butyrophenones (haloperidol)

This is another centrally acting agent. Its main use is in the palliative care setting. It can be given subcutaneously or rectally and so may be helpful if other routes are unavailable. It can be incorporated into syringe drivers if continuous opiate infusions are planned. Haloperidol is given as 2 mg i.m.

Table 35.1 Some causes of nausea and vomiting.

Cause	Example
Mechanical	Bowel obstruction
	Increased intra-abdominal pressure (e.g. ascites/pregnancy)
	Irritative
	Postoperative
Metabolic	Uraemia or electrolyte disturbances
	Diabetic ketoacidosis
	Alcohol
	Malignancy
	Endocrine (e.g. Addison's disease)
Drugs	Opiates and related drugs
	Cytotoxic therapy
	Toxic levels of drugs such as digoxin
CNS causes	High intracranial pressure
	Vestibular disease
	Meningeal irritation
Infective	Gastroenteritis
Psychogenic	Anxiety

CNS, central nervous system.

Antihistamines (cyclizine)

This may be useful in a range of different clinical settings, but is particularly effective for nausea and vomiting with underlying causes such as Ménière's disease and motion sickness. It antagonizes the prokinetic effects of metoclopramide. There may be antimuscarinic effects. Cyclizine 50 mg t.d.s., orally, i.m. or i.v.

5-HT₃ antagonists (ondansetron)

These drugs block receptors both centrally and in the gastrointestinal tract. They are highly effective in postoperative nausea and vomiting and in the alleviation of symptoms associated with chemotherapy and radiotherapy. Dexamethasone is often used synergistically. Give 4 mg orally or i.m., or 16 mg p.r.n.

Dopaminergic blockade (metoclopramide)

This acts centrally and peripherally and has a mild prokinetic effect, aiding stomach emptying. In high doses it can be used as part of a chemotherapy regimen. It has no role in opioid-related nausea. As with the phenothiazines, dystonic reactions may occur. Domperidone has fewer central effects and so is less sedating. It can be used in cytotoxic therapy and in the treatment of drug-induced vomiting of Parkinson's disease. Metoclopramide is given as 10 mg orally, i.m. or i.v., repeatedly to a maximum of 500 micrograms/kg/24 h.

Cannaboids (nabilone)

This has only limited usefulness but is worth trying in the therapy of malignancy or cytotoxic-induced symptoms that have proved resistant to other therapies.

Hyoscine

This may be useful for motion sickness but little else.

These are most commonly seen as a side-effect with the use of phenothiazines or dopaminergic blockers. Young patients (especially females) and the elderly appear to be particularly at risk. These reactions manifest as skeletal and facial muscle spasms and oculogyric crises. They are a consequence of the relative excess of cholinergic activity resulting from the blockade of the dopamine receptors. Treatment should be with an antimuscarinic agent, such as procyclidine 2.5–5 mg orally or benzatropine 1–2 mg i.m. or i.v., repeated if necessary.

Postoperative nausea and vomiting

Anaesthesia can induce severe nausea. An antihistamine (such as cyclizine 50 mg t.d.s. orally, i.m. or i.v.) or a phenothiazine (such as prochlorperazine) are mainstays of treatment. For resistant cases, a 5-HT$_3$ antagonist, such as ondansetron 8 mg preoperatively, can act as prophylaxis. It may be continued at 8 mg at 8-hourly intervals for two more doses.

If vomiting is seen after this period, consider if the operation or its precipitating cause could be implicated. Ileus is common after surgery, not just in those patients who have had an abdominal operation. Electrolyte disturbances, especially hypokalaemia, may contribute to this ileus and severe electrolyte disturbance may in itself trigger vomiting.

Chemotherapy/radiotherapy

Ondansetron and dexamethasone are often part of the therapeutic regimen and the dosage is dependent on how emetogenic the chemotherapy might be.

Opioids

Prochlorperazine and cyclizine are useful. If the opioid is being given for severe acute pain, such as myocardial ischaemia, giving simultaneous antiemetics is prudent.

36: Gastro-oesophageal reflux and peptic ulcer disease

Gastro-oesophageal reflux

Gastro-oesophageal reflux disease (GORD) is caused by the retrograde flow of gastric contents through an incompetent lower oesophageal sphincter causing oesophageal erosions and inflammation. At the mildest end of the spectrum, mild oesophageal inflammation is seen, while in severe cases peptic strictures and intestinal metaplasia (Barrett's oesophagus) can be seen. Barrett's oesophagus is associated with an approximately 30-fold increase in the risk of adenocarcinoma of the oesophagus.

Non-pharmacological management

Assuming a correct diagnosis of GORD, initial treatment should include lifestyle changes. Of principal importance is the need to lose weight, which can be confirmed in most patients by checking their body mass index (BMI). This single intervention may be enough to eradicate most or all of the patient's symptoms. Avoidance of coffee and alcohol, giving up smoking and eating smaller meals (especially late in the evening) may all help. Drug therapy should not be regarded as a means of allowing patients to continue with an unhealthy lifestyle.

Consider also whether any of the patient's existing medications are contributing towards reflux symptoms:

NSAIDs, theophylline, tricyclic antidepressants, ACE inhibitors, calcium-channel blockers, opiates and potassium supplements.

Pharmacological treatment

Antacids

These include aluminium hydroxide, calcium carbonate, magnesium salts and sodium bicarbonate. They are available over the counter and many patients will have tried them prior to seeking medical advice. They produce rapid but brief symptom relief by raising gastric pH. Antacids can alter electrolyte balance and decrease the absorption of iron, vitamin supplements, salicylates, tetracycline and cimetidine.

Alginates

These act by forming an alkaline cap that sits on top of the gastric contents. The rationale is that this both reduces reflux and provides a mechanical barrier for the oesophagus against the reflux of acid contents. Both alginates and antacids may be effective at symptom relief in mild GORD.

Mucoprotective agents

Preparations such as sucralfate act locally by shielding damaged mucosa and stimulating local defence mechanisms via prostaglandin (PG) formation.

Bismuth covers the base of ulcers by forming a glycoprotein precipitate. It has a formidable side-effect profile and is now used less.

Misoprostol is a prostaglandin E1 (PGE1) analogue. It inhibits gastric acid secretion and stimulates bicarbonate production and local blood flow. It is usually used as a combination preparation with NSAIDs (*Arthrotec*). It has significant effects on uterine contractions and so is contra-indicated in pregnancy because of the risk of miscarriage. It is used as part of the medical termination of pregnancy.

H$_2$-receptor antagonists

The histamine$_2$-receptor blockers reduce gastric acid secretion. These are widely prescribed and used. Occasionally, patients report diarrhoea as a side-effect. Dizziness, tiredness, altered liver function tests and gynaecomastia are also sometimes seen. Cimetidine binds to microsomal p450 and so can impair the metabolism of other drugs, such as phenytoin, warfarin and diazepam. Amongst practitioners favouring a step-up policy in the management of GORD, H$_2$-receptor antagonists are normally the next line of treatment in patients not controlled on antacids or alginates.

Proton-pump inhibitors

These drugs inhibit the hydrogen–potassium adenosine triphosphatase of the gastric parietal cell. Their side-effect profile is small: principally rash, headache and, occasionally, diarrhoea. They have a number of interactions with other drugs including warfarin and phenytoin. In symptomatic patients who need to continue taking an NSAID, proton-pump inhibitors (PPIs) or misoprostol (see below) may be useful for prophylaxis.

PPIs are more effective than H$_2$-blockers in maintaining remission of GORD [1]. However, according to NICE guidelines, PPIs should be reserved for severe GORD or for patients in whom the disease is complicated by stricture, ulceration or haemorrhage [2]. Others favour the top-down approach to the treatment of GORD, and start with a PPI and gradually reduce treatment intensity for maintenance as symptoms resolve. Whatever approach is taken, PPIs should be used for maintenance at the lowest effective dose. This drug and other drugs for GORD should be regularly reviewed as they can mask the symptoms of malignancy. Patients with atypical changing symptoms in the older age category should have an endoscopy.

There is probably little to choose between the different PPIs [3]. The important differences are in cost and slight variations in indication. Individual hospital formularies often dictate which PPI should be used. Formulations are tablets or capsules, suspension and now intravenously, although this remains debated (Table 36.1).

Helicobacter pylori infection

Two-thirds of people with *Helicobacter pylori* infection are asymptomatic. However, this bacterium is responsible for most cases of peptic ulcer disease (the other significant cause being NSAIDs). It is also a major risk factor for the development of gastric cancer. Diagnosis may

Table 36.1 Proton-pump inhibitor indications and regimens.

Benign gastric	Benign duodenal	NSAID induced	Relapsing prophylaxis	Nasogastric tube	Intravenous dose
Omeprazole					
20 mg b.d., 8 weeks	20 mg o.d., 4 weeks	20 mg o.d., 4 weeks	10/20 mg	Dispersible tablets, 10, 20 or 40 mg	40 mg
Esomeprazole					
	40 mg o.d., 4 weeks		20 mg	N/A	N/A
Lansoprazole					
30 mg o.d., 8 weeks	30 mg o.d., 4 weeks	15–30 mg o.d., 4 weeks	15 mg	30 mg sachets	N/A
Pantoprazole					
40 mg o.d., 4 weeks	40 mg o.d., 2 weeks		20 mg o.d.	No	40 mg

N/A, not applicable; NSAID, non-steroidal anti-inflammatory drug.

be based on biopsies, usually from the gastric antrum, although infection may be elsewhere in the stomach. These biopsies can be subjected either to histological analysis, culture or urease tests. The sensitivity with any of these tests is approximately 85–95%. Non-invasive tests, including urea breath tests, serology and stool antigen testing, are available.

Peptic ulcer disease

Duodenal ulcer

Amongst patients not taking NSAIDs, *H. pylori* will be the cause of duodenal ulcer in 95% of cases (see above). In uncomplicated cases of duodenal ulcer in patients not on NSAIDs, *H. pylori* eradication should be sufficient to bring about healing (see below). Maintenance therapy with an H_2-blocker or PPI after

H. pylori eradication should not be necessary and, provided that symptomatic relief is complete, repeat endoscopy should not be necessary.

Gastric ulcer

The investigation and management of these ulcers are slightly different because the differential diagnosis of an endoscopically 'innocent-looking' gastric ulcer includes malignancy. Biopsies should be taken from the ulcer prior to starting treatment to allow the diagnosis of *H. pylori* infection. Although the association between *H. pylori* and gastric ulcers is not as strong (approximately 80%) as it is for duodenal ulcers, eradication treatment should be started if infection is confirmed.

In patients with complicated gastric ulcers (a history of haemorrhage or perforation), antisecretory drugs should be continued until after there is endoscopic proof of ulcer healing. All patients with gastric ulcer should have an endoscopy to confirm healing and to allow repeat biopsies from the ulcer site to exclude malignancy.

In patients with gastric ulcers, every effort should be made to reduce the risk factors associated with ulceration. The patient should be encouraged to give up smoking. If possible, the patient should stop taking NSAIDs. If this is not possible, then prophylactic misoprostol 200 micrograms orally 2–3 times daily or a PPI should be used.

Helicobacter eradication therapy

All treatments are based on acid suppression and antibiotics to eradicate the pathogen. The choice of acid suppressant and antibiotic is determined by local policy. However, two examples are given below.

1 Omeprazole 20 mg b.d. orally + amoxicillin 1 g b.d. orally + clarithromycin 500 mg b.d. orally.

2 Omeprazole 20 mg b.d. orally + clarithromycin 500 mg b.d. orally + metronidazole 400 mg b.d. orally (suitable for penicillin-allergic patients).

Treatment is normally for 1 week, with approximately 90% eradication rates. Higher rates may be possible with longer courses, although adverse effects are increased and compliance is reduced. Tests to confirm eradication should be delayed until at least 4 weeks after eradication treatment and at least 2 weeks after cessation of PPIs, as false-negative results may be seen.

Patients with symptoms (duodenal or gastric ulcer) and *H. pylori* infection should be treated with eradication therapy. The screening and/or treatment of asymptomatic patients for *H. pylori* infection is not yet justified by the literature. There is no evidence that this decreases the incidence of gastric cancer.

The role of surgery

Surgery should be considered if symptoms are recurrent or there is Barrett's oesophagus. It may also be used in patients who are PPI dependent and wish to come off treatment. Surgery can be performed as an open or laparoscopic procedure (in skilled hands). Patient selection is important, with surgery tending to be particularly effective for symptoms improved by PPIs. This antireflux surgery rarely, if ever, improves atypical symptoms, such as globus, not improved by PPIs.

References

1 Hallerback B, Unge P, Carling L *et al*. Omeprazole or ranitidine in long-term treatment of reflux esophagitis. Scandinavian Clinics for United Research Group. *Gastroenterol* 1994; **107**: 1305–11.

2 *Guidelines On the Use of Proton Pump Inhibitors in the Treatment of Dyspepsia*. National Institute for Clinical Excellence, UK. Technology Appraisal Guidance No. 7, 2000.

3 Langman MJ. Which PPI? *Gut* 2001; **49**: 309–10.

37: Insomnia, nocturnal confusion and the aggressive patient

General measures

Night sedation is often requested. The old adage that 'if a patient is tired enough, they'll sleep' still pervades some places. It is easy to understand that a worried patient, feverish, generally ill and on a noisy ward with a disrupted night–day cycle might well find it difficult to get to sleep. Sleep is essential and occasionally some pharmacotherapy may be needed.

There are no tight rules governing night time sedation. The aim is often to give enough anxiolysis and mild short-acting sedation to counter the distraction and disturbances of hospital and hence break the cycle of poor sleep, bad day, frustration and poor sleep again, but these drugs should not be given often unless there is a system of regular review (Fig. 37.1).

If a patient is already on a form of night sedation, stopping it acutely is unlikely to do much good unless the acute pathology will be affected. The first question should really be whether the insomnia is a manifestation of night time agitation, excessive stimulants (coffee at bedtime, late prescription for steroids) or depression. Therapy can be tailored accordingly.

Agents used for treating insomnia

Of the common agents used for simple insomnia, the most widely prescribed are the short-acting benzodiazepines, followed by a range of other sedatives and anxiolytics.

Temazepam

Temazepam is a short-acting hypnotic benzodiazepine. It has a half-life of approximately 12 h and no active metabolites. Like all benzodiazepines, it can lead to psychological and physical dependency and should only be given for short durations (under 1 month). If long-term use has occurred, withdrawal must be very gentle. In the elderly, ataxia and confusion may be seen. The common dosage is 10–20 mg 1 h before bedtime. Occasionally, residual hangover effects are seen in the morning and so the regimen should be adjusted accordingly.

Zopiclone

Zopiclone may have fewer hangover effects at lower doses (3.75 mg) but, at high doses and with regular prolonged use, dependency can also be seen. Although not a benzodiazepine, it acts via similar receptors.

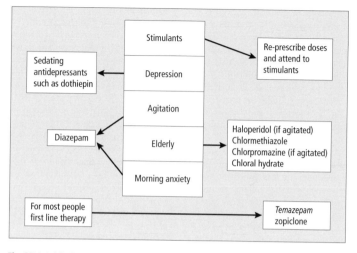

Fig. 37.1 Initiating therapy for insomnia and night time agitation.

Other drugs

In the elderly, thioridazine was often prescribed but it has recently been found to be associated with ventricular rhythm disturbances and so is now limited to second-line therapy in psychoses only. Clomethiazole (192 mg) can also be used here. Haloperidol 2.5–5 mg can be used in the elderly patient with night time agitation.

For suspected depression, the psychiatry service should be consulted; benzodiazepines can often make the symptom worse. For cases related to agitation, chlorpromazine (25 mg) is useful but the question of why there is agitation should be addressed first. Diazepam is more useful to counter early morning waking with agitation. Diazepam has a half-life of up to 20 h and also an active

desmethyl metabolite which can have effects for up to 200 h if given regularly.

Sedation at night is not advised if the acute pathology may be affected, e.g. obstructive sleep apnoea, acute exacerbations of airways disease, head injury and CNS infections. Increased care should be taken of dyspnoeic patients; those who have not slept well can tire quickly and may then deteriorate. Here, less sedating anxiolysis is useful and low-dose paroxetine or trimipramine (25 mg) can be considered.

The violent aggressive patient

Patients are often in hospital because they have actively sought treatment in the majority of cases. There is a tacit agreement to give and receive the best therapy available. However, the patient can refuse therapy at any time and the clinician has to agree to this unless it is felt that the condition is life-threatening and the patient has not made a rational decision. At this point, a range of regulations exist under the law. A patient can be restrained and treated under common law if at immediate danger to himself/herself or others.

At one end of the spectrum is the aggressive patient who is frustrated about something, and communication and explanation are usually all that are needed. In some cases, hospital security teams are needed to emphasize the availability of a quiet place to talk. At the other end of the spectrum are the actively psychotic, proving a danger to themselves and others. Keep yourself, your team and other patients safe. The police can be summoned to assist at any stage and this should be done via the senior nurse. There is also a duty of care to the other patients and it may be necessary to remove the agitated patient from the situation for the overall good. Seek help early. Agitation, confusion and aggression can be a marker for personality type, psychoses, drug-induced or metabolic confusion. A quick review of notes, drug chart, blood results and witness histories can help to establish the cause.

If the patient wants to self-discharge and has a condition that is not immediately life-threatening, is coherent and review has shown an obvious and resolvable trigger, such as alcohol, then he/she should be allowed to go, having first clarified his/her intentions on a self-discharge form. This should be witnessed and the event fully documented. A person has no compulsion to stay in hospital and it should be remembered that people have different priorities. It might be vital for a person to go home to care for a pet, child or parent rather than wait for some pills, so be sympathetic. Discharge medication can be given to a person wanting to self-discharge but this should be fully noted on the GP letter. Usually, only 3 days of medication are given.

If the patient has a history of psychosis, this may be an exacerbation and an acute increase of normal medication may be useful. Look back in the notes to see if this has happened before to tailor response to previous experiences (higher dose, calling a particular family member, etc.).

Pharmacological treatment

If the situation is more volatile, sedation will be needed. Ideally, the negotiated oral route is best and haloperidol 2–5 mg orally is often enough. If this is not possible, physical restraint and forced sedation can be used. When giving any form of forced benzodiazepine sedation, there is a real possibility of overdose and so it is essential that full resuscitation facilities and reversal agents (*Anexate*, flumazenil) are available.

The intravenous route is best as it works fastest and is more predictable than the deep intramuscular route. It may be difficult to site a cannula on a violent patient, so use the easiest and safest route for the first dose; 10 mg haloperidol i.m. or 2–5 mg i.v. can be given as first line. It can be repeated at higher doses after 30 min. Lorazepam 2 mg i.v. is preferable to diazepam 10 mg i.v. as the pharmacokinetics are more predictable. If there is no response, further lorazepam or haloperidol can be used at 30–60-min intervals. If, having used 30 mg of diazepam or 8 mg of lorazepam and 20 mg of haloperidol, there has been no improvement at all, full sedation with anaesthetic support may be needed. At this stage intravenous midazolam or propofol can be considered.

Once a little calm and safety have been achieved, the case should be fully reviewed, looking for triggers and reversible causes. A full set of blood tests should be taken including glucose. Urine toxicology, if possible, is also of use. It is important to establish a diagnosis of some sort here. Does the patient need a CT scan or lumbar puncture? If so, anaesthetic support may be needed.

Regular oral haloperidol, diazepam or lorazepam can be used after this stage. Other forms of therapy should be used as second-line after advice from psychiatric teams. Do not embark on a treatment regimen for medium- or long-term use without this input.

If drug abuse is suspected as the cause of the agitation, such as amfetamines, resins or cannaboids, the situation can be quite fraught. Sedation will almost certainly be needed and, because of the unpredictable nature of the response and the minefield of other systemic effects, close airway and cardiovascular support may be needed. The patient may also need to be placed in a high dependency unit.

38: Drug dependency syndromes

Patients with drug dependency syndromes present with both physical and psychological symptoms. Tachycardia, labile blood pressure, pyrexia and loss of appetite are common. Visual hallucinations, irritability and sleep disturbance can be seen in the more florid cases. The common dependencies encountered are on alcohol, benzodiazepines, barbiturates, nicotine, opiates and amfetamines.

The aim of therapy is to identify the withdrawal, identify the drug of dependency and then try to soften the fall. None of these are easy. The quantity of drug used is less important than the regularity and the duration of exposure for cases of psychological dependence.

Drug treatments

Chlordiazepoxide is the preferred aid to withdrawal as it has less addictive properties and fewer risks of respiratory arrest than chlormethiazole, especially if taken with alcohol. It is safer to give in the discharge and out-patient setting. A typical divided dose regimen for chlordiazepoxide is given in Table 38.1. In severe cases, the dosage and duration of therapy should be increased.

Wernicke–Korsakoff syndrome

This can manifest in chronic alcoholics. Vitamin supplements should be given acutely in those felt to be under-nourished. Intravenous *Pabrinex* can be given. This should be administered before any hyperosmolar fluids or dextrose.

Oral thiamine 300 mg initially then 100–300 mg/day can be given for as long as needed and folic acid and vitamin B complex, two tablets once daily, can also be given.

Opiates

Morphine addiction is becoming increasingly common as is the incidence of those on an active (methadone) withdrawal regimen. The best means of dealing with this situation depends on the facilities available in the hospital. Heroin withdrawal can start within hours of the last dose and symptoms typically peak at around 3 days. Withdrawal from methadone also peaks at around 2–3 days. Occasionally, patients who have had a prolonged exposure to opiates, as in an ITU setting, may show some signs of dependency but these are usually short lived.

It should not be the policy of the hospital to maintain a dependency, but similarly it is unreasonable to suppose that an addict with an intercurrent medical problem can stop overnight. There is a local liaison service that can give advice and often out-reach teams can attend. Patients are not always honest about the amount of heroin consumed, and exaggerating the amount can lead to danger-

Table 38.1 A suggested chlordiazepoxide regimen for withdrawal. It is probably prudent to add 'as required' chlordiazepoxide or diazepam 5–10 mg to the drug chart. Lorazepam may also be useful.

	Morning dose (mg)	Lunchtime dose (mg)	Evening dose (mg)
Day 1	30	30	30
Day 2	20	20	30
Day 3	20	10	30
Day 4	10	10	20
Day 5	10	0	10
Day 6	Stop		

Table 38.2 Methadone equivalent doses of opioids that have been used for recreation/abuse.

Drug	Methadone equivalent
Street heroin	Unclear
Pharmaceutical heroin, methadone, morphine 1 mg	1 mg
Diconal 10 mg	4 mg
Dihydrocodeine pethidine 10 mg	1 mg
Dextromoramide 10 mg	20 mg
Codeine phosphate 300 mg	2 mg
Pentazocine 25 mg	2 mg

ous overdosing. The drugs used in hospital are purer than most available on the street. Street preparations are difficult to define and so any replacement regimen should be titrated to response (Table 38.2).

If the patient is on a treatment regimen for a dependency, consult with the prescribing unit and GP and continue therapy if safe to do so. For a new patient, liaise with the local dependency unit as soon as possible. Withdrawal symptoms should be fully documented in the notes. Examine routes of administration. An estimate of the methadone equivalents used is useful.

Intravenous access can be difficult but important. A compliant patient may be able to indicate accessible veins to establish a line. The initial dose should be 20–30 mg methadone orally. The ideal dose is one that reduces the drug craving to a tolerable level, without sedation or euphoria. Regular half-hourly observations are needed. If symptoms persist, then a further 10 mg can be given after

3 h and repeated as needed. Usually not more than 60 mg are needed in the first 24 h.

On day 2, take the total dosage for day 1 and give this over two or three equal doses. This may need adjustment up or down depending on the response. Further drug may be required and, if this is the case, add 5–10 mg at a time. On day 3, some form of equilibrium should be established and a maintenance level of 50–120 mg/day should be reached. On day 4, the long half-life (>24 h) allows once daily administration but twice daily is safer.

If a previously stable dosage is not adequate, check if the patient has been prescribed or is taking anything that might activate or is inhibit the liver. Alcohol is a very common agent. Benzodiazepines, haloperidol and opioid analgesics used concurrently can worsen CNS depression and should be avoided in the early stages until good control is established. Even then they should be used with extreme caution.

Methadone is a powerful opiate. It has a slow onset of action but a long half-life and can lead to addiction. It is a controlled drug and comes in two formulations: 1 mg/mL and 10 mg/mL. Prescriptions should state the dose in milligrams to be given very clearly. Avoid the use of volumes, as this can lead to confusion. In combination with alcohol and benzodiazepines, there is a high risk of overdose symptoms similar to a general opiate overdose.

Naloxone can be used to correct overdose immediately but, because of its very short half-life, repeat administrations and very close monitoring of the patient are needed. It comes as 1-mL ampoules or a minijet containing 0.4 mg. The usual dosage is 0.4–2 mg over 2 min, which should provoke some improvement. An infusion of 2 mg in 500 mL of normal saline titrated to response may also be needed. Smaller doses can be given if mild respiratory depression is the only feature (1.5–3 micrograms/kg every 2–3 min).

An acute forced reversal is often met with aggression and so precautions should be taken to ensure staff and other patients' safety. Physical restraint of a patient is allowed if he/she is at immediate danger to himself/herself or others. The patient should be discouraged from self-discharging at this time as he/she continues to be at risk.

If the withdrawal regimen is to be continued in the community, the GP and local addiction service must be involved. The discharge provision should be for a GP appointment within 48 h and a meeting with the local addiction group. Prescriptions should not be for more than 3 days.

Nicotine

Nicotine addiction is very common. A life-long smoker with a high level of dependency can manifest with marked withdrawal symptoms as in alcoholics. Nicotine withdrawal is very much overlooked in hospitals. This results in a punitive 'cold turkey' for this legal drug. Nicotine patches and gum are available and should be used if safe. Depending on the working diagnosis, ask if absolute cessation of cigarettes is going to influence management in any great way. Hospital policy has always acknowledged (sometimes unofficially) the need for designated smoking areas for patients and staff alike.

The current NICE guidelines suggest that nicotine replacement therapy (NRT) should only be offered to motivated people who commit to a target cessation date. Therapy should be for 2 weeks only before a further assessment of compliance.

Amfebutamone is an adjunct to motivational support. It has a long list of side-effects but is helpful in a well-motivated group. Its main concern is an increased risk of seizures and it is contra-indicated in those at high risk of seizures.

In acute or severe cardiovascular disease, there are concerns that NRT can make matters worse. It is not advised for use within a few days of an acute infarct or dysrhythmia. It can be used thereafter.

Benzodiazepines

Awareness of the highly addictive properties of benzodiazepines has now restricted their use, but it is still possible to encounter people who have been on regular 20 mg or higher doses of temazepam as a night time sedative for years. A gradual withdrawal regimen is needed and the GP should be made aware of this. All members of this drug class are addictive and so a change in type is rarely successful as a detoxification method. In general, regular benzodiazepines should not be given for more than 2 weeks at a time. At discharge, this should be made clear in the prescription.

In acute toxicity, benzodiazepines can be reversed transiently with flumazenil. This comes as 100 micrograms/mL in 5-mL ampoules. It is given as an intravenous bolus of 200 micrograms over 15 s and repeated 100-microgram doses at 60-s intervals. In head injury cases or in those in whom benzodiazepines have used to treat seizures, rapid withdrawal can precipitate further convulsions.

As with opiates, people with a prolonged hospital stay or a period spent in an ITU setting may manifest benzodiazepine dependency.

Barbiturates

These are now relatively rare as drugs of prolonged abuse. They should only be prescribed in anaesthesia, ITU conditions and intractable insomnia (if already on barbiturates). Phenobarbital can also be used for seizures on rare occasions. The sudden cessation of barbiturates after prolonged use is associated with seizures. A gradual withdrawal is essential.

Other drugs

It is said that an addictive personality will become addicted to anything. In all cases it is important to detect that a withdrawal reaction is occurring. In the acute setting, decide if removal of the drug in question will do more good than harm, then act accordingly.

39: Palliative care and the management of chronic pain

The dying patient is sometimes the hardest to look after. There are issues relating to the patient, family, nursing staff and other members of the medical team. No amount of communication skills seminars will prepare you properly and fully. Your role is not to facilitate or to prolong the dying process but to allow a person to die pain-free and with little physical distress, with the option of loved ones present, in surroundings that are appropriate to that person. This should take into account the religious, cultural and personal view of the patient and family.

Pharmacology has a role in palliative care but should only be viewed as part of the overall care of these patients. There are a number of issues in terminally ill patients:

1 What is the prognosis from the underlying disease and to what extent is the patient (and family) aware of the likely course and timescale of the disease?

2 Does the patient wish for active treatment in the event of clinical deterioration (e.g. intravenous antibiotics for chest infection)? Do the patient and family want resuscitation in the event of a cardiopulmonary arrest?

3 Is discharge to a hospice institution or hospice at home desirable and possible?

Normal medicines

The patient may be taking a large quantity of drugs, which should be reviewed. Aspirin for CVA prophylaxis may not be needed and insulin regimens might be better simplified with less strict glucose control. It may be possible to reduce the pills significantly in consultation with the patient.

Analgesia

Pain is a common feature of terminal disease. The nature of incurable disease results in pain being almost invariably chronic and often progressive. Its successful treatment can improve patients' quality of life immeasurably in their final few days of life.

As with analgesics for acute pain (see Chapter 13), it is sensible to start with simple analgesics, such as paracetamol or NSAIDs, for patients with mild pain. For patients with more severe pain, opiates are second-line therapy. These may be administered in several ways.

Oral aqueous morphine

Oral aqueous morphine has several advantages. It is a powerful analgesic which patients may self-administer. This allows it to be easily titrated against pain without the need for repeated injections.

The starting dose of oral morphine

for a patient previously on large amounts of simple analgesics is approximately 5–10 mg 4-hourly orally. The dosage can be titrated to response. If using large quantities regularly, long-acting preparations should be chosen.

Oral morphine tablets

There are two types of oral morphine tablet. One has similar pharmacokinetics to oral aqueous morphine and should be prescribed in equivalent doses 4-hourly. The second type is slow-release morphine, which need only be taken every 12 h. It is worth considering that some patients prefer tablets to aqueous solutions (although tablets are less suitable for those patients with dysphagia). The slow-release tablets require only 12-hourly dosage and will result in less sleep disturbance.

Once control has been established for 24 h or more with a short-acting version, switch to a sustained release (SR) formulation with a dose interval of 12 h (*MST Continus* or *Oramorph SR*) or of 24 h (*Morcap SR, MXL* capsules). If opiates are used for breakthrough pain, immediate release formulations (*Oramorph*) should be given at one-sixth of the total daily dosage. These should be available as needed. Dosage review and any adjustments to the longer acting agents should be made on a daily basis.

There are several advantages to this type of regimen. Sedation is minimized as analgesia is more tightly linked to pain. The preparations are oral and so the patient is spared from regular injections and may self-administer if this is appropriate. The inclusion of a slow-release morphine preparation decreases the probability of sleep disturbance.

Combined regimens

It is good practice to continue simple analgesics when starting opiates. There is significant adjuvant benefit and they may reduce the need for opiates.

Problems with oral morphine preparations

Constipation

Dietary measures should be instituted as soon as the problem is recognized. If dietary manipulations alone fail, rectal examination should be undertaken to assess faecal loading. If the rectum is full, then two glycerine suppositories are appropriate. For those with an empty rectum, a reasonable food intake but constipation, then a stimulant laxative and/or faecal softener may be appropriate. Co-danthramer two tablets (25/200) *nocte* is commonly employed for this purpose.

Sleep disturbance

Oral aqueous morphine requires the patient to take 4-hourly doses for optimal pain control. This may cause the patient to wake in the middle of the night in pain. If this happens, the patient should take up to twice his/her usual dose at night time. This has useful sedative properties and usually allows the patient to omit the middle of the night dose. An alternative is to prescribe slow-release tablet preparations.

Vomiting and nausea

This may occur as a consequence of

opioid use, but might result from the disease process itself. Prochlorperazine 5 mg 8-hourly orally may be sufficient to control this. More resistant cases may benefit from 8 mg ondansetron 8–12-hourly orally. In patients in whom nausea and vomiting interfere with their ability to take oral medications, the parenteral route can be used for analgesia (see below).

Sedation/confusion and dependence

These are often only transient and may be reduced by using the minimum dosage required to achieve analgesia. An explanation of these symptoms should allay the fears of patients and their relatives. A degree of dependence is common but not normally troublesome in the context of palliation of terminal disease.

Patients in whom oral intake is restricted

Adequate pain control should be possible with the therapies described above, because the dosage can be escalated until analgesia is achieved. However, the oral route may become inappropriate because of coma or confusion, dysphagia or bowel obstruction. There are then a number of available options.

Intermittent parenteral opioid administration

Opiates may be given intramuscularly or subcutaneously. Generally, diamorphine is more suitable than morphine for parenteral administration. It is more soluble and can be given in smaller volumes. However, if the patient has been taking oral morphine preparations, and conversion to parenteral morphine is desired, then this is easily achieved. The *total* parenteral dosage over 24 h is one-half the *total* oral (aqueous and tablet) 24-h dosage. This total parenteral dosage should then be divided by six and given every 4 h.

Conversion to parenteral diamorphine from oral morphine requires a different calculation. The *total* 24-h diamorphine dosage is one-third the *total* oral 24-h morphine dosage. This figure is divided by six and this amount is given 4-hourly.

Parenteral opioid infusion

This may be preferable as it prevents the need for regular injections. Portable pumps are available to aid patient mobility further. These pumps can be used by patients at home although this requires someone, such as a district nurse, to change the syringes approximately every day.

The total 24-h dosage of diamorphine is calculated as for intermittent parenteral diamorphine (i.e. one-third of the 24-h total oral morphine dosage). Subcutaneous infusion via a butterfly needle is an effective means of delivery. The needle should be changed every 24 h. The diamorphine should be dissolved in water. An infusion volume of 0.1–0.3 mL/h is optimal. This determines the amount of water in which the diamorphine should be dissolved. If nausea is problematic, haloperidol 2.5–10 mg/24 h may be added.

Transdermal fentanyl

These are patches applied to the skin and changed every 72 h, providing a sustained release of the opioid fentanyl. Four 'strengths' are available: 25, 50, 75 and 100. These numbers refer to the number of micrograms of fentanyl released per hour, for 72 h, by the patch. Conversion from oral morphine is made by calculating the total 24-h oral morphine dosage. Oral morphine 90 mg in 24 h is equivalent to 25 micrograms/h from a fentanyl patch. The clinical effect of fentanyl patches is not seen until 24 h after starting treatment; during this period, pre-existing analgesics should be phased out gradually as symptoms permit.

Other clinical conditions

Neuropathic pain

This may respond dramatically to tricyclic antidepressants, such as amitriptyline, starting at a dose of approximately 25 mg at night (10 mg in the elderly or frail). This also causes sedation and may aid sleep. Neuropathic pain can also be effectively treated by anticonvulsants, particularly carbamazepine or sodium valproate.

Anxiolysis

Opiates also have an anxiolytic effect. A mild euphoria may ensue. If anxiety persists, then benzodiazepines can be used also. There may be agitation and confusion, depending on the nature of the pathology, which can be treated in the normal way (see Chapter 37). Anti-

psychotics can cause extrapyramidal effects, which may exacerbate a distressing situation, and so their use is probably best limited.

Muscle spasm

Physiotherapy and anti-inflammatory medication help to ease contractures in those with neurological deficits. Muscle antispasmodics, such as baclofen 10 mg b.d. or t.d.s., may also have a role.

Gastrointestinal problems

Gastrointestinal colic benefits from loperamide, although this may exacerbate constipation, which is frequently seen in those on morphine. A starting dose of 2 mg 12-hourly orally is reasonable. Hyoscine hydrobromide 300 micrograms 8-hourly sublingually may also be effective and has a further effective role in drying secretions in those with upper respiratory rattle. The side-effect of dry mouth may limit the usefulness of this drug.

Constipation has already been mentioned as a problem with opiates but may occur as a problem related to the underlying disease process. Its treatment is dealt with elsewhere (see Chapter 34). Lactulose, senna, co-danthramer, enemas and glycerine suppositories may all have a role here.

Malignancy, general systemic upset and medications can all contribute to nausea. Prochlorperazine and cyclizine form the mainstays of therapy. Ondansetron can also be used in resistant cases and is useful in those receiving emetogenic chemotherapy (see Chapter 35).

Nutrition and fluids

A pragmatic view should be taken here. Good nutrition is very important for general physical and psychological health. If the patient is too ill to eat or unable to swallow safely, a decision is needed regarding nasogastric or PEG feeding. Often this is inappropriate. Sometimes a patient may stop eating as a final last choice. The decision-making process should include the patient and family.

Fluid supplementation in a patient unable to sustain adequate oral intake is a little more controversial. If a decision is made to give fluid supplementation, then the subcutaneous route of administration should be considered as an alternative to the intravenous route. Up to 2 L/day of fluid can be given via the subcutaneous route via a small butterfly needle placed in the abdomen or thigh. Normal saline is the best choice; water and 5% dextrose should be avoided as these fluids can lead to damage to the skin. These should be prescribed in the normal fluid section of the drug chart. Fluids may be given via a normal giving set without the need for a pump. As with any line, the position should be changed regularly, with the area of insertion being kept very clean. Such a route of fluid delivery has the additional advantage of being easier to manage in the community by district nurses and thus does not interfere with efforts for the patient to be cared for at home.

Special requests

Alcohol, a cigarette, a favourite food, a massage, shave, hair and make-up are all genuine 'last requests'. Whatever these are, they are not likely to do much harm and may allow a little dignity and self-confidence. It is reasonable to be flexible and local policy should be checked. It is rare that such requests are denied unless in the most inappropriate of cases.

The official line in the *BNF* is that if the medicinal properties of alcohol are needed, flavoured rectified spirit can be prescribed on the drug chart. An alcoholic drink 'for the taste' does not need to be prescribed but it should be clearly noted in the medical and nursing notes why it is being allowed and approximately how much.

Conclusions

Effective palliation of symptoms in terminal care is important. Adequate analgesia should be possible following the guidelines outlined above. Pharmacological management of these patients is only one part of the overall strategy and treatment is optimized by elucidating and addressing the fears and expectations of the patient and family.

40: **Diabetes**

Prescribing insulin or oral hypogly-caemics is only a small part of the therapy for diabetes. Preventing the complications of diabetes, such as cardiovascular problems, diabetic eye disease and neuropathies, is as important. However, the corner-stone of prevention is good long-term diabetic control. Nutrition is very important. Do not restrict car-bohydrate and protein consumption too rigidly. Diabetics can actually become malnourished in hospitals because of fixation on achieving a BM value. A full and healthy diet is more important and that may require a higher dose of hypoglycaemics.

This chapter concentrates on the range of therapies available for the treatment of diabetes, including how to initiate and maintain an insulin regimen. Many related issues are covered elsewhere.

Oral hypoglycaemics

Oral hypoglycaemics work by stimulat-ing insulin release or its peripheral effects. They are used in the treatment of type 2 diabetes and should be reserved for those patients failing to respond to dietary measures and an increase in physical activity. There are a number of different classes of drugs, as shown in Table 40.1.

General principles of use

1 These drugs are used in type 2 diabetics who do not show insulin resistance.

2 Can induce hypoglycaemia (not met-formin), so a source of glucose should always be available.

3 Are best avoided in renal and liver disease.

4 Can cross into breast milk.

5 Should only be given if there will be adequate food intake soon after, so prescribe in-patient regimen to account for local meal times and in-patient procedures.

6 Should be substituted for insulin during a severe illness or if food intake is limited.

7 Start at the lowest dose at the first main meal of the day.

8 Avoid long-acting agents in the elderly.

9 Should be used as part of overall education, lifestyle modification and as-sessment of other risk factors. Patients should be able to recognize hypogly-caemic symptoms and know how to act accordingly.

10 Combination therapy using different classes of drugs can be tried and insulin can be used concurrently.

Sulphonylureas

Sulphonylureas are indicated for type 2 diabetes as monotherapy or in combina-tion with metformin and insulin. They

Table 40.1 Types of oral hypoglycaemic medications.

Drug class	Example
Sulphonylureas	Glibenclamide
Biguanides	Metformin
Insulin secretagogues	Repaglinide
Thiazolidinediones	Rosiglitazone
Alpha-glucoside inhibitors	Acarbose

act predominantly by stimulating insulin release (and thus are dependent on some residual beta islet cell function). Hypoglycaemia can be induced by sulphonylureas and this may persist for many hours. Very close observation is needed in cases of sulphonylurea-induced hypoglycaemia.

The sulphonylureas often encourage weight gain and should only be prescribed in patients who have failed dietary methods of glucose control. They should also be used with caution in patients with hepatic or renal impairment as these patients are particularly at risk of hypoglycaemia.

A range of agents exist with differing half-lives and peripheral effects and are listed in Table 40.2.

Biguanides

Metformin is the only available biguanide. Its mechanism is not entirely clear but it appears to increase peripheral utilization of glucose while reducing gluconeogenesis. It has no direct effect on insulin release and therefore will not induce hypoglycaemia. It has less effect on weight gain compared to other agents.

The results of the recent UK Prospective Diabetes Study (UKPDS) [1] have shown that it is possible to obtain good blood sugar control (as measured by HbA$_1$c) with metformin in overweight type 2 diabetics, with a consequent reduction in diabetic-related complications, deaths and hypoglycaemic episodes, compared to treatment with insulin or sulphonylureas. This has made metformin many clinician's first choice drug for obese type 2 diabetics. In cases where control is poor with metformin alone, insulin or sulphonylureas can be added to the regimen.

The main side-effect is lactic acidosis which can be precipitated in renal failure. The contrast media used during radiological examinations can make renal function worse and so metformin should be avoided for at least 12 h prior

Table 40.2 The different types of oral hypoglycaemics.

Tolbutamide	Short-acting	Can be used in mild renal impairment and in the elderly
Gliclazide	Short/medium duration	Hepatic metabolism so has a use in renal failure, also in the elderly
Glibenclamide	Long-acting	Avoid in the elderly
Glimepiride	Long-acting, newer agent	Possibly less weight gain problems and safer in the elderly
Chlorpropamide	Very long-acting	No longer advised

to and 24 h after any such investigation. It must be used with caution—and preferably avoided—in liver and heart failure. It induces nausea and diarrhoea and should be stopped if the patient is otherwise ill as it may make him/her feel much worse.

Metformin should be prescribed in small doses with meals. The starting dose is 500 mg with breakfast and a step-up by 500 mg with lunch and then dinner. An alternative regimen is 850 mg twice a day. The maximum dosage is 3 g/day, although there is unlikely to be much more benefit at the higher doses. Renal and liver function tests prior to therapy should be available and checked at least twice a year thereafter and after any systemic upset.

Insulin secretagogues

Repaglinide and nateglinide act by increasing insulin release. They have been marketed for those who have irregular meal times, but can also be used as normal therapy or in combination with metformin. Indeed, nateglinide is licensed only for use with metformin. Dosage is adjusted to response. Hypoglycaemia can occur and these drugs should be avoided in liver and renal disease. Like sulphonylureas, they must be avoided in pregnancy and breast-feeding. They should be stopped and substituted by insulin if there is an intercurrent medical problem.

Thiazolidinediones

These are still largely restricted to initiation by specialists. They work by increasing peripheral sensitivity to insulin and are currently licensed for combina-tion therapy with metformin or sulphonylureas. In some countries, this class of drug is also used in combination with insulin. Recent NICE guidelines advocate the use of these drugs for those with inadequate control on metformin/sulphonylurea combination therapy, as an alternative to insulin. However, if the dosage of these drugs was maximal already, insulin production was probably failing and insulin therapy is generally inevitable. Hepatic toxicity has been reported widely and use is to be avoided in those with liver disease. If a patient is admitted on this drug, it is probably useful to move to insulin during the acute phase. It can be reintroduced at a later date. They are often euphemistically and incorrectly called 'glitazones'.

Alpha-glucoside inhibitors

Acarbose is an inhibitor of intestinal alpha-glucosidase, an enzyme involved in the breakdown of complex carbohydrates. It retards the glucose uptake from the small bowel and so attenuates the postprandial peaks in plasma glucose. The resultant increase in colonic carbohydrates leads to a fermentation-like effect with a consequent increase in bowel gas and flatulence. It can be used on its own or in combination with other drugs.

Diabetic ketoacidosis

Diabetic ketoacidosis (DKA) is a medical emergency and carries significant mortality if not addressed early. There are four main components to treatment:

1 Correction of fluid deficit.

2 Provision of insulin.
3 Correction of electrolyte imbalance.
4 Concurrent treatment of any acute precipitating event or sequelae.

Correction of fluid deficit

The aetiology of the fluid deficit in diabetes can be many and varied. It includes the osmotic diuresis secondary to high plasma glucose. Fluid resuscitation should be aggressive. Normal saline should be used initially, until the plasma glucose falls below 15 mmol/L, then move to using 5% dextrose. The first litre of fluid should be given in under 30 min. Fluid replacement may be helped by using central access and CVP monitoring. A urinary catheter may also be useful.

Provision of insulin

Constant low-dose intravenous infusion of short-acting insulin should be used. A peripheral line is adequate for this.

Make a solution of 50 units of soluble insulin up to 50 mL with saline (equivalent to 1 unit/mL). This is given via a syringe and titrated according to a sliding scale regimen. A dose of 6–10 units is given acutely intravenously, followed by a constant infusion. The scheme provided in Table 40.3 is a guide only. A patient with very high insulin requirements needs higher doses and the scale should be adjusted appropriately. The hospital may have separate prescribing sheets for insulin but, if not, write it on a separate fluid prescription chart. Every insulin solution syringe sometimes needs to be individually prescribed.

If intravenous access is difficult, deep

Table 40.3 A suggested insulin sliding scale.

Blood glucose (mmol)	Rate of insulin infusion (unit/h)
0–4.0	0–0.5
4.1–7.0	1
7.1–11.0	2
11.1–17.0	3
17.1–24.0	4
> 24.1	Call doctor

intramuscular injection of 20 units of soluble insulin acutely is acceptable.

Correction of electrolyte imbalance

Insulin induces a net movement of potassium into cells. The resultant hypokalaemia can lead to cardiac rhythm problems. The plasma potassium should be checked twice a day and supplements given to maintain it at approximately 4–5 mmol/L. This may require as much as 250 mmol potassium in the first 24 h. Significant dehydration and possible underlying renal disease may make potassium homeostasis precarious. Potassium can be given as a separate infusion but this requires central access and it is more simply given peripherally by addition to the fluid bags at 40 mmol/L.

The use of bicarbonate is controversial. It is usually reserved for severe decompensating acidosis (pH < 6.9). It should be given in the context of aggressive resuscitation and then only as 100 mL of 8.4% sodium bicarbonate (equivalent to 100 mmol) over at least 30 min through a large vein and repeated as needed.

Treatment of concurrent illness

The only available history of the unwell patient with DKA may be from the patient's family. Compliance with medications and evidence of intercurrent illnesses should be sought by direct questioning. These may also be found from clinical examination. Consider broad-spectrum antibiotics if infection seems likely. If the patient has a decreased conscious level, then consider a nasogastric tube to prevent aspiration. Gastric stasis is seen and the patient should be kept nil by mouth during the acute episode.

Moving from an intravenous to a subcutaneous regimen

A simple method is to take the total insulin used over 24 h of a normal diet and give this in divided doses as a mixture of short- and intermediate- or long-acting preparations (Table 40.4). This is the standard basal bolus practice. A patient previously established on insulin is likely to have similar requirements again.

Long-acting insulins can take up to 14 h to have maximal effect, with a decay that may last up to 24 h. For this reason it is advisable to start them with the sliding scale still running. Mixed preparations

can also be started in this way but with a reduction in intravenous insulin and close monitoring for hypoglycaemia. Short-acting insulins have a peak effect around 2 h after subcutaneous injection. They should be given 20–30 min prior to a meal. This allows high plasma insulin values to correspond to postprandial blood sugar peaks. In NHS hospitals, an evening meal is served around 6 p.m. and so the prescription should take this into account. Getting the patient to self-medicate is very useful and this should be encouraged with the help of a specialist nurse if available.

Intermediate-acting insulins start to work within 2 h and have a peak effect at 4–6 h from injection. Their effects last around 12 h. When using these, the levels will have fallen by about 3 a.m. if given at 5 p.m. and this is likely to result in higher pre-breakfast BMs. This can be dealt with by shifting the evening intermediate dose to later on, or using a long-acting agent instead.

Biphasic insulins are made up as combination products with short and medium duration of action. They are generally written as the product name with the ratio of the insulins noted, e.g. *Mixtard 30* is 30% soluble insulin and 70% isophane insulin, and *Humulin M5* is 50% soluble insulin and 50% isophane.

Most insulin preparations are re-

Table 40.4 Types of insulin preparations.

Insulin	Chemical properties	Peak effect (h)
Short-acting	Soluble	2
Intermediate-acting	Isophane or zinc suspension	4–6
Slow onset, long-acting	Crystalline insulin zinc suspension	12

combinant human analogues, although porcine and bovine versions still exist. There should be no difference in the efficacy of the pure products but combination therapy and mixing short and medium agents in the same syringe may lead to problems. If starting insulin afresh, use human analogues.

The prescription chart should have a short-acting insulin available on the p.r.n. side with instructions of how much to give and at what BM values. *Hypostop* (10 g glucose as a gel), 10% or 50% glucose intravenously should also be available to deal with hypoglycaemia.

The goal of treatment is to achieve good control of blood glucose with minimal impact on patient lifestyle and to avoid episodes of hypoglycaemia.

If initiating therapy in otherwise stable patients for whom DKA is not the precipitating event, the dosage can be started low with 5 units of short-acting insulin subcutaneously 20 min prior to every meal. There is often some recovery of endogenous insulin secretion in the early months and insulin requirements may reduce during this 'honeymoon period', although requirements usually increase again. Combination therapy using the various insulin preparations would be the next step and this should be performed with the help of the local diabetes team and specialist nurses.

In patients with type 2 diabetes who require insulin, the insulin regimen can often be easily managed with twice daily injections of a premixed insulin containing short- and medium-acting insulins. In older patients, diabetes may be adequately controlled by a single daily injection of a long-acting insulin.

Do not expect to obtain a perfect regimen at the first prescription. Patient variability, exercise, concurrent illness, diet and type of insulin all have a role and there is often a long gestation time for an ideal regimen.

Points on the prescribing of insulin

• Short-acting agents 20 min before a meal.
• Medium-acting agents with the morning short-acting drug.
• Long-acting insulin in the evening, at or soon after the evening meal.

Combination biphasic insulins can be used and these are chosen once an equilibrium is established.

Allow for mid-morning, mid-afternoon and supper snacks if possible. Hourly checks of blood sugar are not necessary in the vast majority of cases. A pre-meal check is useful and a 2-h postprandial check will catch most problems. Waking a patient with otherwise good control and no new problems at 4 a.m. to carry out a blood sugar test is inappropriate. The target blood sugar is between 4 and 7 at rest, allowing a transient rise up to 10 soon after a meal. If the value is too high or too low 2 h after a meal, reduce or increase the relevant short-acting agent (Table 40.5). Check what kind of meal the patient received and whether it was appropriate.

Snacks are useful in some contexts but excessive intake can create problems. The dietitian should be involved in a review of nutritional needs. If the blood sugar levels are very volatile, compliance, area of injection, intercurrent disease and quality of the insulin should be reviewed. The area of injection

Table 40.5 Method for altering basal bolus regimen.

Check time	Blood glucose too high	Blood glucose too low
Before breakfast	↑ Evening long-acting agent	↓ Evening long-acting agent
Before lunch	↑ Morning short-acting agent	↓ Morning short-acting agent or consider a mid-morning snack
Before dinner	↑ Pre-lunch short-acting or morning medium-acting agent	↓ Pre-lunch short-acting or morning medium-acting agent. Mid-afternoon snack?
Before bed	↑ Evening short-acting agent	↓ Evening short-acting agent or allow a supper snack
Early morning	Move evening long-acting agent times or check if there is excess night time snacking	A slight reduction in evening long-acting agent may be enough

should be changed regularly to avoid local fat necrosis.

If a very tight control is needed, as in acute MI or in sepsis, then an intravenous sliding scale should be employed.

Discharge of patients on insulin or oral hypoglycaemics

In patients started on insulin in hospital, on discharge they should be given their insulin, graduated 1-mL syringes and needles, a sharps bin and a needle cutter if giving fixed needle and syringe combinations. Patients will need to monitor their own blood glucose and should be given a finger-pricking device, reagent strips for blood sugar monitoring and urine analysis or an electronic meter and test strips. A booklet can also be given to record blood sugar values. For patients on oral hypoglycaemics, drug administration is simpler although these patients also need monitoring equipment.

Non-ketotic hyperosmolar state

In this state, severe hyperglycaemia can occur without significant ketosis. It may be precipitated by the consumption of excessive amounts of glucose, intercurrent illness or triggered by the use of medications such as steroids.

Dehydration is the prominent feature. The extent of insulin deficiency may be less severe than that in DKA. Treatment mainstay is fluid resuscitation with much smaller quantities of insulin being needed. Subcutaneous heparin for DVT prophylaxis should be given.

Hypoglycaemia

This can be seen in cases of high metabolic activity, such as sepsis, and when insulin or oral hypoglycaemics have been used at a dosage greater than subsequent glucose intake. Treatment depends on the cause but, initially, need be no more complicated than giving the patient some sugar, a glass of milk or a sweet drink. There are some more specialized treatments including 10 g of glucose as a gel (*Hypostop*), which is applied to the buccal mucosa.

If intravenous access is already present, 10–20 mL of 50% glucose followed by an infusion of 10% glucose is indicated. This should be given into a large vein as it can be very irritant. If the cause of the hypoglycaemia is an overdose of sulphonylureas, the effects may continue for days and very close monitoring is needed with a constant glucose infusion during that time. In cases where severe hypoglycaemia occurs with loss of consciousness and there is no intravenous access, glucagon can be given (1 mg i.m., i.v. or s.c.). When patients in the community are at risk of hypoglycaemia, carers and family should be instructed on how to use these agents.

The surgical patient with diabetes

The management of diabetes in the perioperative stage has to be simple and safe. The aim is to maintain good blood sugar control but not to deny carbohydrates and so prevent a catabolic state. The differences in prescribing depend upon the previous insulin needs of the patient if any, type of surgery and intercurrent problems.

Type 2 non-insulin-dependent diabetes mellitus

For minor procedures, the patient should be on a morning list as early as possible. Breakfast is omitted as are the morning oral hypoglycaemics. These should be restarted with the next normal postoperative meal. Antiemetics should be given routinely and if there is significant postoperative vomiting, then the glucose, potassium and insulin (GKI) regimen, as below, can be used until symptoms settle.

For poorly controlled NIDDM or more complex procedures, the patient should be admitted at least 24 h prior to the operation so that he/she can be stabilized on insulin therapy. This can be as a sliding scale infusion or the GKI regimen. After the operation, normal medications can be reintroduced when eating normally.

For insulin-dependent patients, a period of 24–48 h in hospital prior to the operation is useful to establish good glycaemic control. Omit long-acting insulins 24 h prior to surgery. If the operation is in the morning, omit the morning insulin dose and omit breakfast; if it is in the afternoon, a light breakfast and short-acting insulin can be given. The GKI infusion can be started in the morning (after breakfast if appropriate) and continued postoperatively until the normal diet resumes. This is not designed for long-term use and, if it is needed for more than 2 days, it is more appropriate to start a formal sliding scale infusion of insulin with fluid containing dextrose and added potassium as needed.

For larger operations, more supplemental fluid may be needed; a dextrose bag is largely water and so is not ideal replacement fluid. In this case, a more rigid sliding scale insulin infusion regimen is needed with a separate dextrose and potassium infusion. Aim for a BM of between 6 and 11 in this group. This may be needed for some time and normal subcutaneous insulin can restart when the patient is on a normal diet. The method of restarting this is as for the DKA patient above.

In some hospitals, the GKI protocol appears to be used whatever the aetiology of poor control, even DKA. As long as there is regular monitoring of blood sugars this should still be safe but it is good practice to give dextrose-free fluid and insulin in the early stages until the BM is below 15 mmol/L.

The GKI regimen

The glucose, potassium and insulin (GKI) regimen is designed to provide a continuous supply of carbohydrate in the form of glucose, potassium replacement and insulin to an otherwise stable patient. This allows for a more protected metabolic state during the perioperative period when the patient would otherwise be starved. It requires a 1–2-hourly BM check and the ability to change the infusion type regularly if needed.

Bag 1: 500 mL of 10% dextrose + 10 mmol of KCl + 15 units of short-acting insulin.
Bag 2: 500 mL of 10% dextrose + 10 mmol of KCl + 20 units of short-acting insulin.
Bag 3: 500 mL of 10% dextrose + 10 mmol of KCl + 10 units of short-acting insulin.
Start with Bag 1 and check BM after 1–2 h. If BM < 6, move to Bag 3 and recheck after 1 h. If it is still below 6, stop the infusion for an hour. If BM > 11, move to Bag 2 and recheck after 1 h.

Reference

1 Effect of intensive blood-glucose control with metformin on complications in overweight patients with type 2 diabetes (UKPDS 34). UK Prospective Diabetes Study (UKPDS) Group. *Lancet* 1998; **352**: 854–65.

Appendix: Sample prescription form

The following sample prescription form gives examples of sections found in most hospital prescription forms.

Generic General Hospital NHS Trust
Prescription and Administration Record

(Space for patient identification label)

Date of admission	3 / 4 / 20 03
Date of planned discharge	/ / 20

TTOs written	TTOs received by pharmacy

Name (Surname) NOTHER	Unit No. 0123456	
First Names ANN	DOB 10/4/1945	
Consultant		
Ward 6H	Site	
Height . . .150. . . . . . . cm	Weight . . . . .65. . . . . . kg	
House Officer ADOC	Bleep 1234	

Chart Number 1 of 1

Allergies, Drug Intolerances and other useful information
ELASTOPLAST – CONTACT DERMATITIS
MIGRAINE INDUCED BY CAFFEINE

Notes to prescribers

Write legibly in black ink and use approved names for all drugs (Except where trade names are essential).

Please avoid use of decimal point where possible.

Any changes in drug therapy must be ordered by a new prescription, DO NOT alter existing instructions.

This prescription sheet is valid for two weeks only.

Antibiotics:

Review IV antibiotics after 24 hours.

The IV route should be changed to oral as soon as clinically possible.

Please indicate a stop date when initiating oral treatment.

Pre-medication, Once only drugs and Prophylactic Antibiotics

Date	Time	Drug	Dose	Route	Signature	Given			Pharmacy
						Date	Time	Initials	
4/4	0800	TEMAZEPAM	10 mg	O	ADOC				
				induction					
4/4 on induction		CEFUROXIME	1.5 g	IV	ADOC				
4/4		METRONIDAZOLE	500 mg	IV	ADOC				
4/4	0800	BRUFEN	800 mg	O	ADOC				

Oxygen Therapy

Drug Oxygen Low concentration (Venturi Connector)			Date					
Concentration 24/28/31%	Frequency (Delete*) PRN* or Continuous*		Time					
Target saturation	Signature	Start date	Given by					
Drug Oxygen Low concentration (Nasal cannulae)			Date					
Rate 1–4 litres/min	Frequency (Delete*) PRN* or Continuous*		Time					
Target saturation	Signature	Start date	Given by					
Drug Oxygen Medium to High concentration			Date					
Rate 4–15 litres/min	Frequency (Delete*) PRN*		Time					
Target saturation 95%	Signature ADOC	Start date 4/4	Given by					

When required medication

Drug				Date					
Dose	Frequency	Route	Start date	Time					
Additional instructions			Pharmacy	Dose					
Signature				Route					
				Given by					

Infusion Therapy

Each prescription is once only. A new prescription must be written if the infusion is repeated

Date	Infusion solution	Additives and dose	Volume	Rate	Route	Doctors's signature	Time started and stopped	Added by and given by	Pharmacy
4/4	N/SALINE		IL	6Y˙	IV	ADOC	0800 1400	AN AN	
4/4	N/SALINE	+ 20mmol KCl	IL	8Y˙	IV	ADOC			
4/4	GELOFUSINE		500mls	STAT	IV	ADOC			

Regular Medication

Notes to nursing staff

When a drug is NOT administered, record the appropriate number and your initials, in the relevant box and if appropriate document in the nursing records:–

1. Patient away from ward
2. Patient could not take drug or supplement (e.g. Nil by mouth, Vomiting)
3. Patient refused drug or supplement
4. Drug or supplement not available
5. Nursing decision (document in nursing records)
6. On instructions of doctor (document in nursing records)
7. Patient is self-administering medication or supplement
8. Not all drug or supplement taken

Warfarin at 6pm		Date							
Target INR/Indication	Start date	INR							
		Dose							
Signature	Pharmacy	Sig.							
		Given by							

			Date / Time	4/4	5/4						
Drug PARACETAMOL			06 –	X							
Dose 1g	Frequency qds	Route O	Start date 4/4	12 –							
Additional instructions		Pharmacy	18 –								
Signature ADOC			24 –								
Drug BRUFEN			08 –	X							
Dose 400mg	Frequency tds	Route O	Start date 4/4	14 –							
Additional instructions with food		Pharmacy	22 –								
Signature ADOC											
Drug CEFUROXIME			06 –	X							
Dose 1.5g	Frequency tds	Route IV	Start date 4/4	14 –							
Additional instructions		Pharmacy	22 –								
Signature ADOC											
Drug METRONIDAZOLE			06 –	X							
Dose 500mg	Frequency tds	Route IV	Start date 4/4	14 –							
Additional instructions		Pharmacy	22 –								
Signature ADOC											

Blood/Blood Components/Blood Products

Date	Type of Blood/ component/ product	CMV Neg Yes/No	Irradiated Yes/No	Volume	Rate	Doctor's Signature	Unit/Batch No.	Time started & stopped	Checked by and given by
4/4	PACKED RED CELLS	N	N	1 unit	4̇	ADOC			
	FFP			1 bag	20 min	ADOC			

PCA and Epidural Prescriptions

				Syringe 1	Syringe 2	Syringe 3
Patient Controlled Analgesia			Date started			
Drug 1 & amount added MORPHINE 50mg	Drug 2 & amount added		Time started			
			Signature			
Diluent & syringe volume N/SALINE 50 mls	Loading dose NONE	Route IV	Checked			
			Date stopped			
Background infusion NONE	PCA Bolus dose 1 mg	Lockout time 5 min	Time stopped			
			Stopped by			
Follow PCA guidelines, DO NOT GIVE OTHER SYSTEMIC OPIOIDS WHILST ON PCA						
Naloxone	Dose 400 mg	Route IV	Date			
If respiratory rate " 8 per minute, or patient unrousable			Time			
Signature ADOC	Date 4/4	Pharm.	Given by			

				Syringe 1	Syringe 2	Syringe 3
Epidural Analgesia			Date started			
If epidural opioids administered, Do not give systemic opioids			Time started			
Drug 1 & Concentration	Drug 2 & Concentration		Signature			
		Route	Checked			
Diluent & syringe volume	Infusion rate		Date stopped			
			Time stopped			
Naloxone	Dose	Route IV	Date			
			Time			
If respiratory rate " 8 per minute, or patient unrousable			Given by			
Ephedrine	Dose	Route IV	Date			
If required for severe or persistent hypertension			Time			
Signature	Date	Pharm.	Given by			

Index

Page numbers in *italics* indicate figures; those in **bold** indicate tables.

Notes